POSTSTROKE DEMENTIA AND IMAGING

POSTSTROKE DEMENTIA AND IMAGING

V. MOK, W. W. M. LAM, Y. L. CHAN AND KA SING WONG

Nova Biomedical Books
New York

For permission to use material from this book please contact us:
Telephone 631-231-7269; Fax 631-231-8175
Web Site: http://www.novapublishers.com

Library of Congress Cataloging-in-Publication Data

ISBN 978-1-60692-247-7

Available upon request

Published by Nova Science Publishers, Inc. ; New York

Contents

Preface

Stroke increases the risk of dementia by approximate 2-9 times. World wide, vascular dementia (VaD) is the second commonest cause of dementia. Presence of poststroke dementia (PSD) reduces survival among stroke survivors and increases risk of long term stroke recurrence. Varying severity levels of cognitive impairment affects functional outcome independent of physical impairment. With an aging population, burden of PSD is expected to rise. Although PSD is prevalent, relevant to mortality and morbidity, and is potentially more preventable than Alzheimer's disease (AD), it has received less attention relative to poststroke physical impairment or to AD. It is not until the last decade that more attention has been paid to PSD.

Historically, in the late 19th century, VaD was considered to be the commonest cause of dementia. It was thought that dementia was due to a relentless strangulation of the brain's blood supply, resulting in degeneration of the brain and dementia. In the middle of the 20th century, pathological studies have begun to reveal that senile plaques and neurofibrillary tangles, rather than vascular lesions, were key findings among most of the elderly demented patients with atrophic brains. In the early 70s, VaD was thought to be uncommon and the mechanism of VaD was attributed to multiple small or large cerebral infarcts (multi-infarct dementia). In recent decades, advances of neuroimaging have enhanced greatly our understanding on VaD, its complexity far exceeds that of the concept of multi-infarct dementia. The authors aim to review the current understanding of PSD and its imaging. Poststroke dementia will first be defined. Following that, foundational issues of PSD including its classification, pathology, prevalence, and cognitive pattern will be reviewed. This sets the background for discussing the imaging aspects relevant to PSD.

A. Introduction

Stroke increases the risk of dementia by approximate 2-9 times [1-5]. World wide, vascular dementia (VaD) is the second commonest cause of dementia [6-7]. Presence of poststroke dementia (PSD) reduces survival among stroke survivors and increases risk of long term stroke recurrence [8-10]. Varying severity levels of cognitive impairment affects functional outcome independent of physical impairment [11-14]. With an ageing population, burden of PSD is expected to rise. Although PSD is prevalent, relevant to mortality and morbidity, and is potentially more preventable than Alzheimer's disease (AD), it has received less attention relative to poststroke physical impairment or to AD. It is not until the last decade that more attention has been paid to PSD.

Historically, in the late 19th century, VaD was considered to be the commonest cause of dementia. It was thought that dementia was due to a relentless strangulation of the brain's blood supply, resulting in degeneration of the brain and dementia [15]. In the middle of the 20th century, pathological studies have begun to reveal that senile plaques and neurofibrillary tangles, rather than vascular lesions, were key findings among most of the elderly demented patients with atrophic brains. In the early 70s, VaD was thought to be uncommon and the mechanism of VaD was attributed to multiple small or large cerebral infarcts (multi-infarct dementia) [15]. In recent decades, advances of neuroimaging have enhanced greatly our understanding on VaD, its complexity far exceeds that of the concept of multi-infarct dementia [16,17]. We aim to review the current understanding of PSD and its imaging. Poststroke dementia will first be defined. Following that, foundational issues of PSD including its classification, pathology, prevalence, and cognitive pattern will be reviewed. This sets the background for discussing the imaging aspects relevant to PSD.

B. Defining Poststroke Dementia

Dementia comes from the Latin word, *de mens*, which means "without mind". In general, it refers to deterioration of cognitive abilities that are severe enough to interfere daily activities. Various sets of diagnostic criteria for dementia have been proposed over the decades. The most commonly used criteria worldwide are the various editions of the Diagnostic and Statistical Manual of Mental Disorders (DSM) and the International Classification of Diseases (ICD). Albeit emphasis of each set of criteria varies slightly, they share similar framework that requires 3 elements: (1) memory impairment; (2) impairment of one or more cognitive domain, e.g. executive dysfunction, aphasia, apraxia, or agnosia; and (3) the cognitive impairment is severe enough to interfere social functions, such as work or social activities.

In this review, PSD is defined as the presence of dementia noted after stroke, irrespective of presence of preexisting dementia, prior stroke history, mechanisms for dementia, or the latency between stroke and onset of dementia. Stroke is commonly defined according to the World Health Organization as rapidly developing clinical signs of focal (or global) disturbance of cerebral function, with symptoms lasting 24 hours or longer or leading to death, with no apparent cause other than vascular origin. Since majority of the recent studies have evaluated the presence of dementia at 3 months poststroke, those studies that have evaluated dementia longer than 3 months poststroke will be described as delayed PSD in this review [3,18,19]. Most studies on PSD have used various editions of DSM or ICD to define dementia poststroke.

Table 1. Diagnostic criteria for vascular dementia

1a. Hachinski Ischemi Score	
Features	Score
Abrupt onset	2
Stepwise deterioration	1
Fluctuating course	2
Nocturnal confusion	1
Relative preservation of personality	1
Depression	1
Somatic complaints	1
Emotional incontinence	1
History of hypertension	1
History of strokes	2
Evidence of associated atherosclerosis	1
Focal neurological symptoms	2
Focal neurological signs	2

Score > 7 = VaD, score <4 = AD

1b. The NINDS-AIREN criteria
Probable VaD (include all of the following)
1. Dementia = cognitive decline manifested by impairment in memory + 2 or more other cognitive domains that are severe enough to interfere daily activities independent to physical deficits related to stroke
2. Cerebrovascular disease (CVD) = a. Presence of focal signs on neurological examination, such as hemiparesis, lower facial weakness, Babinski sign, sensory deficit, hemianopsia, dysarthria, etc. consistent with stroke (with or without history of stroke); AND b. Evidence of relevant CVD by brain imaging (CT or MRI) including multiple large-vessel strokes or a single strategically placed infarct (angular gyrus, thalamus, basal forebrain, PCA or ACA territories), as well as multiple basal ganglia and white matter lacunes or extensive periventricular white matter lesions or combinations thereof.
3. A relationship between the above two disorders, manifested or inferred by the presence of one or more the following: a. onset of dementia within 3 months following a recognized stroke; b. abrupt deterioration in cognitive functions; or fluctuating, stepwise progression of cognitive deficits

Table 1. Diagnostic criteria for vascular dementia (Continued)

Possible VaD
1. Dementia (as above) + 2a. Focal neurological signs in the absence of imaging confirmation, OR 2b. absence of clear temporal relationship between dementia and stroke, OR 2c. subtle onset and variable course (plateau or improvement) of cognitive deficits and evidence of relevant CVD

1c The ADDTC criteria for ischemic vascular dementia
Probable ischemic VaD (include all of the following)
1. Dementia = decline of intellectual function sufficient to interfere broadly patient's usual daily activities, which is not isolated to a single narrow category of intellectual performance
2. Evidence of two or more ischemic strokes by history, neurological signs, and/or neuroimaging studies (CT or T1-weighted MRI); or Occurrence of a single stroke with a clearly documented temporal relationship to the onset of dementia
3. Evidence of at least one infarct outside the cerebellum by CT or T1-weighted MRI
Possible ischemic VaD
1. Dementia (as above)
2a. A history or evidence of a single stroke (but not multiple strokes) without a clearly documented temporal relationship to the onset of dementia; or 2b. Binswanger's syndrome (without multiple strokes) that includes all of the following: (i) early-onset urinary incontinence not explained by urologic disease, or gait disturbance (e.g. parkinsonian, magnetic, apraxic, or "senile" gait) not explained by peripheral cause, (ii) vascular risk factors, and (iii) extensive white matter changes on neuroimaging

1d. The DSM IV criteria (include all of the following)
1. Dementia=decline in memory impairment + one or more domain of cognitive impairment that cause significant impairment in social or occupational functioning
2. Focal neurological signs and symptoms (e.g. exaggeration of deep tendon reflexes, extensor plantar response, pseudobulbar palsy, gait abnormalities, weakness of an extremity) or laboratory evidence indicative of cerebrovascular disease (e.g. multiple infarctions involving cortex and underlying white matter) that are judged to be etiologically related to the disturbance

Table 1. Diagnostic criteria for vascular dementia (Continued)

1e. Criteria for subcortical vascular dementia (include all of the following)
Cognitive syndrome including both: a. Dysexecutive syndrome: impairment in goal formulation, initiation, planning, organizing, sequencing, executing, set-shifting and maintenance, abstracting b. Memory deficit (may be mild): impaired recall, relative intact recognition, less severe forgetting, benefit from cues c. Which indicate deterioration from a previous higher level of functioning and are interfering with complex (executive) occupational and social activities not due to physical effects of cerebrovascular disease alone
Cerebrovascular disease including both: a. Evidence of relevant cerebrovascular disease by brain imaging (see table 4b) b. Presence or a history of neurological signs as evidence for cerebrovascular disease such as hemiparesis, lower facial weakness, Babinski sign, sensory deficit, dysarthria, gait disorder, extrapyramidal signs consistent with subcortical brain lesion(s)

Poststroke dementia is a broader phenomenon than VaD. The current usage of VaD refers to patients whose dementia is wholly or at least partially attributed to cerebrovascular disease (CVD). Various sets of diagnostic criteria for VaD have been proposed over the decades (table 1), including the Hachinski Ischemic Score (HIS) [20], DSM IV [21], ICD-10 [22], State of California Alzheimer's Disease Diagnostic and Treatment Centers (ADDTC) [23], and the National Institute for Neurological Disorders and Stroke with the Association Internationale pour la Recherche et l'Enseignement en Neurosciences (NINDS-AIREN) [16]. The presence of dementia and evidence for CVD (e.g. history of stroke, focal neurological signs, neuroimaging evidences of CVD) are 2 key elements of these criteria. Most criteria also emphasize evidences for the relationship between CVD and dementia, e.g. dementia onset within 3 months of stroke, abrupt or stepwise cognitive deterioration, fluctuating course, or neuroimaging features that are relevant to dementia. Supporting features for and suspicious features against the diagnosis for VaD are also included in some of the criteria [16, 23]. As will be discussed later, specific imaging criteria have also been incorporated into some of these criteria [16]. Note that not all patients with VaD have history of overt stroke. Overall, these criteria identify different frequencies and clusters of patients [16] with varying sensitivity and specificity [16]. The NINDS-AIREN criteria are probably the most stringent and specific (80%), yet least sensitive (58%) [24, 25], while the DSM IV criteria are the most liberal [24]. Terms such as "probable", "possible", "mixed", or "definite" VaD have been used in various criteria to describe the certainty of which the dementia is attributed to CVD [16,23]. In general, definite VaD requires pathological verification. Recently, diagnostic criteria have also been proposed for a subtype of VaD (subcortical VaD) for use in clinical trials (table 1e).

Given that it is the most prevalent and homogeneous subtype of VaD, recent authorities have suggested that future clinical trials should focus on this entity, rather than mixing various subtypes of VaD together [26]. These criteria are modified from NINDS-AIREN criteria, which put greater emphasis on executive dysfunction and lesser emphasis on the presence of stroke history because executive dysfunction in subcortical VaD may be prominent and overt stroke episode may not occur in subcortical VaD [27]. Note that in these criteria cognitive deterioration that is severe enough to interfere "complex" or "executive" occupational and social activities is already sufficient to fulfill the severity requirement for dementia. Specific imaging criteria are also included in this set of criteria. The specificity and sensitivity of this set of criteria await further evaluation from pathology study.

Different to VaD, PSD refers to presence of dementia noted after stroke that may or may not be attributed to stroke or CVD. Dementia post stroke may be due to other dementing illnesses, e.g. AD. Vascular dementia may be considered as a subtype of PSD. In this review, PSD will be emphasized, yet studies on VaD that have included stroke patients will also be covered.

Note that stroke affecting specific brain regions can induce cognitive impairment that is restricted only to a particular cognitive domain, such as aphasia, apraxia or agnosia [28, 29], or is subtle [30]. The cognitive profile of these cases may not fulfill the standard diagnostic criteria for dementia either because the spectrum of affected cognitive domains is not broad enough or the impact of cognitive symptoms to social function is not severe enough. Although failure to recognize cases with poststroke cognitive impairment that falls short of dementia may underestimate the full impact of CVD or may hinder application of potential preventive treatment [31], for the purpose of this review, this category will not be emphasized.

C. Classification of Poststroke Dementia

To date, a consensus on the clinical classification of PSD that is derived from its mechanisms and is also relevant to its management is not available mainly because its exact mechanisms are yet uncertain. It is currently believed that PSD may involve complex interactions between vascular etiologies, brain lesions, brain atrophy, co-existing dementing diseases and the host factors [17]. The classification framework will certainly evolve as we gain better understanding on the mechanisms of PSD. At present, we propose to classify PSD according to the vascular etiology and the etiology for dementia.

Vascular Etiology

The vascular etiology of PSD includes both "stroke-related" and "concurrent" vascular etiology. Stroke-related vascular etiology covers present or previous stroke(s). Concurrent vascular etiology covers vascular etiology that may explain non-stroke related vascular lesion, e.g. arteriosclerosis that contributes to white matter changes (WMC) or vascular etiology that explains "silent" infarct. Similar to stroke etiology, the vascular etiology of PSD can be classified into large artery disease, small vessel disease (SVD), cardioembolism, miscellaneous causes, hemorrhage, and PSD of undetermined vascular etiology.

Table 2. Classification of poststroke dementia

1. Vascular etiology (stroke-related or concurrent vascular etiology)	
Subtypes	*Brain lesions associated with the vascular etiology*
a. Large artery disease	cortical / large subcortical territorial infarct borderzone infarct (anterior, posterior, superior, internal), lacunar infarct
b. Small Vessel Disease	
lipohyalinosis	lacunar infarct (smaller)
atherosclerosis	lacunar infarct (larger)
arteriosclerosis	WMC
c. Cardioembolism	cortical / large subcortical territorial infarct (frequently multiple), borderzone infarct (anterior, posterior, superior, internal), lacunar infarct
d. Hemorrhage, e.g.	
SVD related	deep (along territory of deep penetrating artery)
cerebral amyloid angiopathy	superficial or lobar
e. Miscellaneous, e.g.	
CADASIL	lacunar infarct, WMC
hemodynamic	borderzone infarct
cerebral amyloid angiopathy (non-hemorrhagic)	lacunar infarct, WMC
f. Undetermined etiology	Variable
2. Etiology of dementia	
a. Poststroke VaD	The dementia is secondary to the stroke and/or concurrent vascular etiologies; current diagnostic criteria for probable VaD can be applied; e.g. of poststroke VaD are subcortical VaD or strategic infarct dementia
b. Poststroke mixed dementia	The concurrent presence of AD that explains mostly or partially the dementia syndrome poststroke
c. Poststroke other dementia	The concurrent present of other non-vascular and non-AD related dementia syndrome, e.g. frontal temporal dementia, dementia with Lewy bodies

1. Large Artery Disease

Large artery disease refers to atherosclerosis affecting extra or intracranial large artery. In Caucasians, it commonly affects extracranial carotid artery, while in Asians, Blacks, and Hispanics, it commonly affects intracranial large artery, in particular, middle cerebral artery (MCA) [32]. Types of brain lesions associated with extracranial carotid atherosclerotic disease are heterogeneous, and may include cortical territorial infarct, large subcortical infarct, borderzone infarct (internal, anterior, posterior, superior borderzone) and even lacunar infarct. Although brain lesions associated with MCA atherosclerotic disease are similar to that with carotid artery stenosis, our recent study demonstrated that the former was associated more commonly with subcortical lacunar infarcts, which were often scattered as chain-like fashion along the internal, anterior or posterior borderzone [33]. If the infarct hits at "strategic" areas or is of adequate size or frequency, it may induce PSD. Strategic area refers to cerebral cognitive eloquent area, which if it is affected, will cause cognitive impairment. Examples of "strategic" areas are thalamus, angular gyrus, genu of the left internal capsule, left anterior corona radiata, anterior corpus callosum, inferior medial temporal lobe, hippocampus, frontal lobe, and caudate nucleus [34-37]. Less commonly, large artery disease may involve multiple arteries sequentially, inducing multiple brain lesions, and result in multi-infarct dementia.

2. Cardioembolism

Emboli from the heart are frequently large, causing impaction at intracranial large artery, resulting in extensive cortical territorial infarct. Scattered emboli may occlude multiple or bilateral arteries simultaneously, inducing multiple large infarcts. Or that recurrent embolic stroke occurs at different times, causing cumulative large brain lesions. The end results of multiple large infarcts may again be multi-infarct dementia. Note that as in large artery disease, types of brain lesions associated with cardioembolism are also heterogeneous, including lacunar infarcts, large subcortical infarct or borderzone infarcts. If infarct hits at strategic areas or is extensive or multiple, dementia may result (figure 1).

3. Small Vessel Disease

Small vessel disease is used here to include only the commonest types of small artery pathologies that are most prevalent among the elderly with vascular risk factors. These include lipohyalinosis (or complex SVD), arteriosclerosis (or simple SVD) and the small vessel variant of atherosclerosis (microatheroma). Other vascular etiologies, e.g. amyloid angiopathy, which also affect small vessels, will not be classified as SVD here. Small vessel disease affects both deep and superficial long penetrating arteries that supply the subcortical and brainstem regions. The brain lesion associated with lipohyalinosis or atherosclerosis is lacunar infarct that is located in the subcortical or brainstem region. Brain lesion associated with arteriosclerosis is WMC, which are located in the deep white matter or periventricular region. White matter change is commonly referred as "leukoaraiosis", where "*leuko*" is "white" and "*araiosis*" means rarefaction. Since present imaging modalities and techniques are not able to visualize small artery lesions, SVD in vivo is diagnosed by presence of radiological lacunar infarcts and/or WMC in the absence of large artery disease, cardioembolism and other miscellaneous causes. Note also that it is only lacunar infarct that is related to overt stroke episode, while arteriosclerosis and WMC are not directly responsible for the stroke event. Although arteriosclerotic related WMC are most prevalent in lacunar stroke, it also exists in other stroke subtypes.

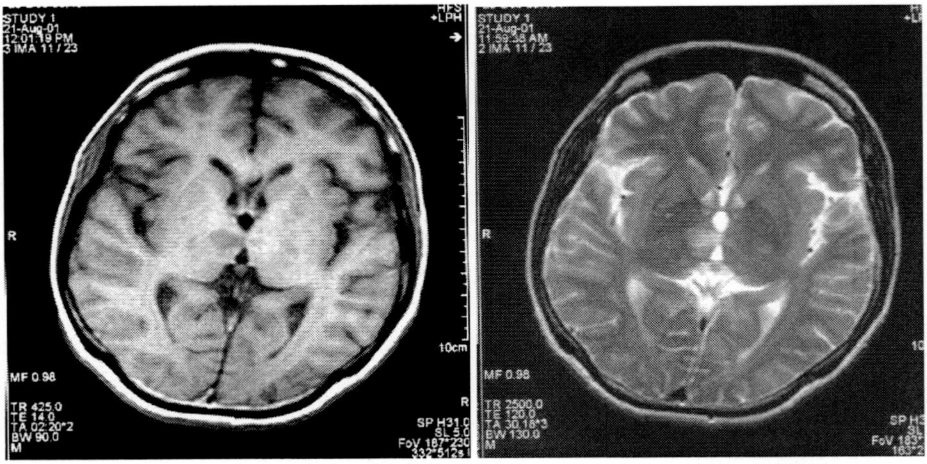

1a. T1-weighted MRI 1b. T2-weighted MRI

Figure 1. Strategic infarct dementia secondary to cardioembolic stroke

A 45-year-old female presented with acute confusion, gaze palsy, and fluctuating consciousness without motor problems. MRI shows bilateral paramedian thalamic infarcts (hypointense on T1- [figure 1a] and hyperintense on T2-weighted [figure 1b] imaging, the left sided lesion is smaller and appears more subtle than the right one; smaller infarcts are also noted lateral to the paramedian thalamic infarcts). Investigation revealed underlying apical hypertrophic cardiomyoapthy and paroxysmal atrial fibrillation. At 3 months poststroke, she remained apathetic along with memory complaints and poor attention span. Her MMSE was 25/30 then. The cognitive impairment affected her daily functioning as a housewife. This case represents a cardioembolic stroke (vascular etiology) causing multiple infarcts at strategic areas (bilateral thalamic infarcts), resulting in a dementia syndrome that has a strong component of executive dysfunction. Both the history and MRI fulfill the NINDS-AIREN criteria for probable VaD.

Binswanger's disease [38] and lacunar state (état lacunaire or lacunar dementia) [39] are probably the commonest examples of SVD that are associated with dementia (figure 2). Brain lesions characteristic of Binswanger's disease are diffuse WMC, yet sparing the U fibers; while that of lacunar state, are multiple lacunar infarcts. Although it has been considered as two distinct entities historically, authorities have recently believed that they are varying manifestations of the same disease [40]. Subcortical VaD has been used to describe these 2 entities collectively. Apart from the above more severe forms of SVD, focal SVD inducing an isolated lacunar infarct that is located in a strategic area, such as genu of the internal capsule, caudate or thalamus, can also induce PSD in the absence of diffuse SVD [35-37].

4. Hemorrhage

In this review, hemorrhagic stroke refers only to intracerebral hemorrhage (ICH). Although subdural, epidural and subarachnoid hemorrhages are all related to dementia, these non-ICH related hemorrhages will not be discussed in this review. Perhaps the commonest form of ICH in the elderly is associated with SVD and hypertension. The brain lesion is usually located in the "deep" cerebral or cerebellar region. If hemorrhage occurs at strategic area, such as thalamus, cognitive impairment or dementia may result [41, 42]. Size of the haematoma or presence of ventricular extension may affect severity of cognitive impairment [41]. Yet, concurrent vascular etiology (e.g. SVD) and brain lesions (e.g. WMC and lacunar infarcts) can also contribute to the dementia syndrome. Cerebral amyloid angiopathy (CAA) affects small artery and has particular relevance to PSD. It is commonly associated with recurrent "superficial" lobar hemorrhages and dementia [43]. The lobar hemorrhage in CAA classically occurs in the absence of hypertension among elderly patient. It is also found commonly in patients with AD. Rarely, CAA is associated with hereditary cerebral hemorrhages. However, the mechanism for CAA related ICH in inducing dementia is complex. Apart from the direct effect of recurrent cerebral hemorrhages, CAA may induce dementia due to concurrent AD and/or its associated concurrent brain lesions, namely WMC and lacunes [44, 45]. Other forms of ICH may include iatrogenic (e.g. warfarin related) and less commonly, arteriovenous malformations, intracranial venous thrombosis or microangiomas. In general, its relevance to PSD is related to the site, size and extent (ventricular extension) of the haematoma.

5. Miscellaneous Vascular Etiology

Miscellaneous subtypes of vascular etiology mainly comprise of rare forms of stroke disorders or CVD. Typical brain lesions may be associated with these diseases. Vascular etiologies of these miscellaneous subtypes of PSD can be further classified into hereditary, e.g. cerebral autosomal dominant arteriopathy with subcortical infarcts and leukoencephalopathy (CADASIL) [46], non-hemorrhagic form of CAA, autoimmune vasculitis (e.g. systemic lupus erythematosus), hemodynamic (e.g. hypoxic-ischemic encephalopathy, severe heart failure, orthostatic hypotension, post-coronary artery bypass graft) or hypercoagulable state, e.g. antiphospholipd syndrome.

6. Undetermined Vascular Etiology

Poststroke dementia of undetermined vascular etiology refers to case where extensive imaging and laboratory evaluations reveal no vascular etiology that can account for the stroke. Patients are commonly young, free of vascular risk factors, having stroke related cortical or large subcortical infarct(s). In many cases, the mechanism is presumed to be embolic in nature as angiography fail to reveal intra or extracranial large artery disease. Yet, cardiac investigation is also unrevealing. Stroke with unknown vascular etiology was found to be associated with PSD [47, 48].

Etiology of Dementia

In a patient with PSD, after determining the vascular etiology and brain lesion, the second step is to determine how much does the vascular related brain lesion contribute to the dementia syndrome poststroke, or in other word, is to determine the etiology of dementia. Dementia after stroke may not be related to stroke or other vascular related etiology and brain lesion, but may be related to other dementing illnesses, e.g. AD. A simple way is to classify etiology of dementia into “poststroke VaD”, “poststroke mixed dementia” and “poststroke other dementia”.

1. Poststroke Vascular Dementia

Poststroke VaD refers to dementia that is predominantly attributed to the stroke or other concurrent vascular etiologies and related brain lesions. However in practice, establishing this causal link between dementia and stroke or CVD is complex and consensus on the methods in doing so has not been reached. In principle, the occurrence of new onset cognitive deterioration poststroke [5, 48, 49] and/or presence of relevant radiological vascular related brain lesions suggest a strong vascular contribution. Relevant brain lesions include infarcts located at strategic sites, multiple territorial infarcts, or multiple lacunar infarcts associated with severe WMC. Many studies have used current diagnostic criteria of VaD as mentioned previously to classify poststroke VaD [11, 50] and imaging criteria defining relevant brain lesions have also been proposed. These criteria will be discussed in detail later. In poststroke VaD, the dementia syndrome can be the direct result of one stroke, the cumulative effects of multiple strokes (multi-infarct dementia), and/or the effects of other concurrent non-stroke related vascular etiology and related brain lesions, e.g. WMC or silent infarcts.

2. Poststroke Mixed Dementia

Poststroke mixed dementia refers to the concurrent presence of AD in a stroke patient with dementia. In daily practice, it is clinically determined by a diagnosis of AD prestroke or a history of progressive prestroke cognitive impairment in the absence of relevant radiological cerebral vascular lesions, e.g. extensive WMC or multiple silent lacunes, which probably already exist prestroke. In mixed dementia, the index stroke episodes may or may not worsen the cognitive impairment poststroke. Information regarding the prestroke cognitive status is usually obtained through closed informants of patients. Instrument such as the Informant Questionnaire on Cognitive Decline has been commonly used to evaluate objectively the presence of prestroke cognitive impairment or dementia [19, 51, 52]. Mixed dementia also covers case where progressive cognitive decline develops poststroke in the absence of further stroke and / or new relevant vascular related brain lesions. In such case, concurrent AD is implicated. Recent studies have shown that vascular brain lesions (e.g. lacunar infarct) may also interact synergistically with Alzheimer's pathology in aggravating the cognitive severity of patients with Alzheimer's pathology [53, 54].

3. Poststroke Other Dementia

The last subtype of PSD is poststroke other dementia. It refers to the presence of other non-vascular and non-AD related dementing illness (e.g. dementia with Lewy bodies or chronic alcoholism) that either exists already prestroke or develops poststroke, and may or may not contribute to the dementia poststroke. In general, other dementia among patients with PSD is rare [48].

In summary, we propose a 2-step classification for PSD, i.e. first, to determine the stroke-related and/or concurrent vascular etiology, second, to determine how much the vascular component, or other dementing illnesses contribute to the dementia syndrome (i.e. etiology of dementia). In clinical practice, determining the etiology of dementia is probably the most difficult. However, attempt to classify PSD according to etiologies based on all available clinical data is still worthwhile as potential effective treatment and prevention rest on accurate knowledge on these aspects of PSD. To date, recent clinical studies have suggested that response to cognitive treatments vary according to vascular etiology and/or etiology for dementia. For example, effects of memantine or nimodipine may be better for subcortical VaD relative to that for large arterial related cortical VaD [55, 56], while acetylcholinesterase inhibitor may be more effective in mixed dementia over probable VaD [57].

D. Pathology of Poststroke Dementia

The role of pathology in diagnosing and classifying PSD in conjunction with clinical information is less concrete than that in AD, where definite pathological markers (neuritic plaques and neurofibrillary tangles) exist [58]. At present, there is no consensus for the pathological diagnosis of PSD [59] and controversies regarding brain substrates that are representative of poststroke VaD remain. Yet, pathology still plays the definitive role in providing information on the presence, nature and extent of vascular lesions, brain lesions, brain atrophy and other concurrent pathologies, e.g. AD, which is relevant in the overall evaluation of PSD. It has been used as the gold standard to evaluate the validity of various clinical diagnostic criteria for VaD.[25, 60] Further pathological studies will certainly contribute in unraveling the mechanisms of PSD. Furthermore, with the advances of imaging techniques, more types of pathological lesions can now be visualized by imaging, which are previously not detectable by standard imaging modality. Hence, understanding the pathological lesions for PSD provide an important interface for interpretation of imaging findings or development of new imaging techniques.

In general, the size (large artery or penetrating small artery), site, types (e.g. atherosclerosis, arteriosclerosis, lipohyalinosis, amyloid angiopathy), and extent of the arterial pathologies are important in the evaluation of PSD. Relevant brain lesions include cortical or large subcortical territorial infarct, borderzone infarct, lacunar infarct, microinfarct, perivascular space, hemorrhage, cortical laminar necrosis, granular atrophy, microbleed, WMC, hippocampal sclerosis, brain atrophy, and other non-vascular related pathologies, e.g. Alzheimer or cortical Lewy bodies pathology [59, 61, 62]. The location, size, extent, and interaction of these lesions may affect its relevance to the dementia syndrome poststroke. The pathology related to PSD has been reviewed recently in detail.[63] A brief overview on key pathological substrates will be presented below.

Lacunar Infarct

Pathologically, lacunar infarct refers to small cavity of size between 3-15mm, which is associated by either in-situ SVD (i.e. atherosclerosis or lipohyalinosis) or embolism from proximal sites causing occlusion of small vessels. Atherosclerosis affects small artery of size 200-800μm and induces larger lacunar infarct (>5mm) due to occlusion [64]. Lipohyalinosis affects arteries of size 40-200μm and may cause smaller lacunar infarct (3-7mm) possibly by occlusion and endothelial leakage associated with breakdown of blood brain barrier (BBB).[64, 65].

Perivascular Space (Virchow-Robin Space)

Similar to lacunar infarct, perivascular space is also a cavity, which is commonly smaller than that related to lacunar infarct. It surrounds a penetrating artery and various hypotheses explain its occurrence, including brain atrophy, mechanical stress from the pulsatile arterioles, or interstitial fluid drainage disorder [64]. Imaging differentiation between lacunar infarct and perivascular space will be discussed later.

White Matter Changes

White matter refers to myelinated axons and glial cells that are located in the deep and periventricular region. Long superficial and deep penetrating arteries originated from the superficial pial plexus and major intracerebral large arteries respectively supply the cerebral white matter. Given that the arteries are long and anastomoses are minimal or absent between deep and superficial penetrators, white matter region is vulnerable to hypoperfusion.

White matter changes describe both ischemic and non-ischemic related white matter pathology. Ischemic WMC consist of pallor of myelin, loss of oligodendrocytes, myelins and axons, cavitation with or without lipid-laden macrophages, and astrogliosis but without definite necrosis [63]. Arteriosclerosis is invariably found in these areas. Note that the strip of white matter that is located just beneath the cortex (U-fiber) is usually spared due probably to adequate perfusion by unaffected shorter vessels located adjacent to the cortex. The cause of the ischemia can be multi-factorial, which may include narrowed arteries related to arteriosclerosis, reduced cerebral blood flow (e.g. cardiac failure, severe carotid artery stenosis), hyperviscosity (e.g. hyperglycemia, polycythemia, hyperlipidemia) and/or impaired cerebral autoregulation [40] The WMC may also be due to endothelial leakage from artery secondary to BBB dysfunction as a result of SVD [65]. Furthermore, study has demonstrated that WMC may be indirectly due to impaired venous drainage associated with collagenous thickening affecting parenchymal veins or venules [66]. In general, ischemic WMC are visualized radiologically as confluent deep WMC or irregular / extending periventricular WMC [67].

Non-ischemic WMC refers mainly to the periventricular spongioform zone that is associated with paucity of myelin, disrupted subependymal lining, and gliosis [67]. The cause for it is probably due to altered periventricular fluid dynamics, which may simply be age-related with no pathological significance. On MRI, these pathological changes are seen as thin rim of caps or smooth halo [67]. Note that small punctate deep WMC shown on MRI might not be visible on autopsy specimens and hence pathological nature of these WMC are uncertain [67].

Microinfarct

Microinfarct ranges from a few microns to 0.5mm and is characterized by loss of myleinated fibers in white matter or total loss of neurons in gray matter. Recent pathology studies have highlighted its relevance to PSD [59, 61]. At present, it cannot be visualized on current imaging modality.

Granular Cortical Atrophy

It consists of multifocal cortical microinfarcts accompanied by focal gliosis, which are commonly found in the cortical borderzone between MCA and anterior cerebral artery. Cerebral hypoperfusion is implicated as the mechanism. Although cortical atrophy may be seen on imaging, identifying microinfarcts by current imaging is not yet possible. Hence granular cortical atrophy associated with microinfarcts remains a pathological diagnosis.

Cortical Laminar Necrosis

Cortical laminar necrosis describes a particular pattern of severe ischemic injury that is characterized by an extensive band of necrosis along cortical layers most vulnerable to ischemia. It is commonly related to hypoxic ischemic encephalopathy associated with global cerebral hypoperfusion or hypoxia.

Hippocampal Sclerosis

Hippocampal sclerosis in the elderly is characterized by severe neuronal loss and gliosis in the CA-1 and subiculum region of the hippocampus, with relative sparing of other hippocampal fields. It is currently believed to be due to ischemia secondary to systemic hypoperfusion or intrinsic CVD.

Microbleed

Microbleed is characterized by hemosiderin around abnormal small vessel, with infarction of the surrounding tissue. Although it was once thought to be silent, a recent study using T2*-weighted gradient-echo (GE) magnetic resonance imaging (MRI) demonstrated its cognitive relevance among stroke patients independent of other ischemic lesions [68].

In principle, poststroke VaD is defined by the presence of relevant cerebral vascular lesions associated with no or minimal plaques or tangles,25, 60 while mixed dementia is defined as concurrent presence of both vascular related brain lesions and significant Alzheimer's pathology [63]. However, as mentioned before, consensus on detailed criteria regarding vascular related brain lesions related to VaD has not been reached.

E. Frequency, Incidence, and Clinical Determinants of Poststroke Dementia

Hospital-Based Studies at Three Months Poststroke

The frequency of PSD in general (i.e. including those with prestroke dementia and prior stroke) at 3 months poststroke based on more recent hospital-based studies ranges from 20% – 32%.[5, 48-50, 69-71]. The frequency of new onset dementia poststroke at 3 months ranges from 9% – 16%, [50, 72] which is around half of that of PSD in general. If only patients with first ever stroke were included, the frequency ranges from 13%-29%, [49, 71, 73] which is slightly less than that of PSD in general. The frequency of PSD after hemorrhagic stroke is probably similar to that of ischemic stroke [69]. The frequency of PSD among different stroke subtypes varies only slightly, [48] although one study revealed that SVD increased PSD by 2.7 times relative to other stroke subtypes [70]. One must also aware that the frequency of PSD also varies with the set of diagnostic criteria that are used to define dementia. In a study among the same cohort of patients, frequency of PSD varied from 6% by ICD-10 to 25.5% by DSM-III [74].

Various clinical and imaging determinants interact to produce PSD. Imaging determinants will be discussed in a later section and the former will be discussed now. Various hospital-based studies have yielded somehow similar clinical determinants of PSD based on multivariate regression analyses. Basic demographic determinants include old age, [2, 5, 48, 50, 69, 70, 72, 73, 75] low education, [2, 5, 49, 50, 70] and non-white population [2, 48, 70] Vascular risk factors predicting PSD include diabetes [48, 70, 73] atrial fibrillation, [5, 69, 75] and prior stroke [5, 48, 49, 70, 72] Stroke-related clinical features that determine PSD include aphasia [5, 49, 73, 75], major hemispheric stroke syndrome, [48, 49, 70] and stroke severity according to clinical scale [50, 69, 72]. Relevant stroke features include left sided cerebral infarct [5, 48, 70, 72] and MCA infarct [50, 73]. Prestroke cognitive and functional impairment also predict PSD [50, 69, 75].

Delayed Poststroke Dementia

Cumulative incidence rate of new onset delayed PSD according to hospital-based studies ranges from about 16% at 1 to 2 year [47, 75] to around 20%-30% at 3 to 4 year [18, 19]. The relative risk of incident dementia associated with stroke as demonstrated by an early study was 3.83 [4]. A recent study found that VaD accounted for two-thirds of delayed PSD at 3 years follow up [19]. In another recent study, the PSD etiology was found to shift from predominantly AD with CVD type (mixed dementia) in the first 2 years and to VaD type later on [18].

Hospital-based incident studies have identified the following clinical determinants for delayed PSD: old age, [3, 4, 18, 19] low education, [3] diabetes mellitus, [19] previous stroke, [47] cerebral hypoxia associated with intercurrent medical illnesses, e.g. cardiopulmonary arrest, cardiac arrhythmias or epilepsy, [4] stroke severity at admission, [19] baseline intellectual function, [3] and prestroke cognitive impairment [19] Most of these factors are similar to that found in hospital-based studies of PSD at 3 months.

Community-Based Studies

Few community-based studies have investigated the incidence of delayed PSD. An earlier study found that the cumulative incidence rate of new onset delayed PSD increased from 7% at 1 year to 48% at 25 year poststroke [76]The incidence of dementia in the first year was 9 times greater than expected and age, male sex, and second stroke were found to predict PSD based on multivariate model [76]. In another community study, incident rate of stroke related dementia was 21.3% at 2 years of follow up and elevated levels of low-density lipoprotein were associated with risk of stroke-related dementia [77]. In the more recent community-based Framingham study, stroke was found to double the risk of dementia relative to controls who were free of stroke and dementia [1]

Interestingly, factors associated with lower risk of AD, namely young age, high education, and presence of 2 apolipoprotein E ε3 alleles, were found to predict delayed PSD. These findings highlight the long-term cognitive consequence of stroke, as stroke appears to nullify the lower prestroke risk of dementia among those with low risk for dementia.

F. Cognitive Pattern of Poststroke Dementia

Different to AD, which has a unique cognitive pattern and progression; cognitive profile of PSD varies with its subtypes and sites of the brain lesions.

Cognitive Pattern with Cortical Brain Lesions

Cognitive pattern of poststroke VaD associated with cortical brain lesions depends on the site of the lesion, and at times, the pattern may be "patchy". For example, cognitive impairment secondary to cardioembolism that induces multiple cortical infarcts involving mesial temporal lobe, dominant frontal-parietal lobe, and medial frontal lobe may present with amnesia, aphasia, ideomotor apraxia, and executive dysfunction. If non-dominant frontal-parietal cortex is affected, dressing apraxia, constructional apraxia, or agnosia may result. A classical Gerstmann's syndrome (agraphia, acalculia, right-left disorientation, finger agnosia) may result if the dominant parietal lobe (angular gyrus) is involved.

Cognitive Pattern with Subcortical Brain Lesions

Subcortical infarcts affecting strategic areas, such as paramedian and polar region of the thalamus, caudate, inferior genu of the internal capsule, and anterior corona radiata commonly produce amnesia and executive dysfunction. The mechanism whereby lesions at subcortical structures produce amnesia and executive dysfunction is probably due to disruption of the frontal–subcortical or medial temporal limbic circuits [78].

Cognitive pattern of poststroke subcortical VaD typically has predominant executive dysfunction. The stroke-related physical deficits commonly include various lacunar syndromes, namely pure motor stroke, pure sensory stroke, ataxic hemiparesis, or hemiballism/chorea/athetosis. Other associated features of subcortical VaD may include urinary symptoms, mood disturbance (e.g. depression), parkinsonism, and gait abnormality [26].

Executive Dysfunction in Poststroke Vascular Dementia

Recent study by Sachdev et al found that executive dysfunction was the predominant feature of poststroke VaD in general and was thought to be related the high prevalence of WMC in patients with poststroke VaD [11]. This study suggested that while large cortical infarcts do contribute to the dementia pattern, they are best regarded as being superimposed on a background of executive dysfunction in those with poststroke VaD [11].

Executive dysfunction refers to a set of loosely related cognitive functions that serve the purpose of coordinating higher order cognitive capabilities and emotion and regulating behavioral responses to environmental demands. It was originally described in patients with frontal lobe injuries, and later in those with subcortical lesions, probably related to disruption of various frontal-subcortical circuits [79]. Features of executive dysfunction may include impaired decision making, poor judgment, distractibility, emotion instability, failure to inhibit inappropriate response, failure of set-shifting, perseveration, poor initiation, poor abstraction, abulia, restricted emotion, deficient empathy, lack of planning, or executive memory loss. Executive memory loss describes memory loss that is due to defective retrieval mechanism, which is different to amnesia in AD, which is due to impaired encoding mechanism related to hippocampal lesion. Patients with executive memory loss will have better recognition memory when cues are given to help memory retrieval, whereas recognition memory remains poor in AD patients [80].

Cognitive Progression in Poststroke Dementia

As mentioned before, poststroke VaD can be the result of a single stroke event or the cumulative effects of recurrent strokes and/or other vascular related brain lesions. The cognitive progression can be acute deterioration poststroke followed by recovery, [81] stepwise deterioration after recurrent strokes, [82] slow progressive deterioration, [83] fluctuating, or any combinations of the above. In general, the cognitive decline in patients with poststroke VaD is slower than those with AD but is faster than those without dementia poststroke [83].

G. Imaging in Poststroke Dementia

Imaging has revolutionized our understanding and management of PSD. At the most elementary level, imaging helps to ascertain the presence of cerebrovascular lesions and to rule out surgically treatable dementias, e.g. subdural hemorrhage, tumor, or hydrocephalus. With the recent advances and availability of various imaging techniques, knowledge on the mechanisms of how vascular etiologies, brain lesions and other brain pathologies interact in producing PSD has been enhanced. A better knowledge on its mechanisms has shaped our present conceptual framework in classifying and diagnosing PSD, and in turn, imaging features have been incorporated into various diagnostic criteria for VaD [16, 26, 84].

Apart from the evaluation of the mechanisms and diagnosis of PSD, imaging has also been proved useful in clinical studies for PSD. In a recent multi-center drug study for probable VaD as defined by NINDS-AIREN criteria, besides fulfilling the criteria for having evidence of dementia, CVD, and the relationship between the two, fulfillment of specific imaging criteria based on MRI as confirmed by a blinded central reader was also essential for inclusion [85]. Given that accuracy of clinical judgment may vary with centers, imaging criteria probably provide the most objective mean to ensure the accuracy in diagnosis.

As will be discussed later, certain imaging features can be used as a prognostic indicator for cognitive progression [86] and have helped in providing insights for therapeutic interventions [87]. It has also been recently hypothesized that progression of WMC as shown by MRI, may help not only to reflect disease progression, but also to act as a surrogate marker in clinical trials on cerebral SVD [88].

H. Basic Imaging Modalities and Methods in Poststroke Dementia

The type of imaging modalities and methods that are used in PSD depends first, on its ability in detecting and quantifying cerebral abnormalities that are relevant to PSD; and second, on the availability and expertise of the individual center. To date, the following imaging characteristics are found to be relevant to PSD: (1) type and distribution of the arterial lesions; (2) type, size, site, and number of vascular related brain lesions (e.g. hemorrhage, stroke-related infarct, borderzone infarct, silent infarct or WMC); (3) severity and distribution of cerebral atrophy (e.g. cortical, subcortical or regional atrophy); (4) severity and pattern of cerebral blood flow, glucose metabolism, and oxygen metabolism; and (5) cerebral vasoreactivity. In this section, imaging modalities and methods that have been used most commonly in practices or researches of PSD will be described.

These include computed tomography (CT), MRI (T1-, T2-, and proton density [PD] weighted, and fluid attenuation inversion recovery [FLAIR]), SPECT, PET, and xenon CT. Since the present clinical diagnostic and classification framework of PSD or VaD are based on findings from structural CT and the above MRI techniques, its methods in the evaluation of PSD will be described first (table 3). The last 3 modalities have been used mainly in research setting and a brief overview on the functions and findings of these standard functional imaging modalities will be given next. The physics and technical details of these imaging modalities are beyond the scope of this review. Following this section, imaging determinants and imaging criteria that are based on the above imaging modalities for PSD will be described respectively. Recent imaging applications on PSD (e.g. diffusion weighted imaging [DWI], diffusion tensor imaging [DTI], magnetization transfer imaging [MTI], T2*-weighted GE sequence, MR perfusion, and MR spectroscopy [MRS]) will be presented last. Although we recognize the importance of angiography techniques (digital subtraction angiography and CT and MR angiography) in the evaluation of vascular etiology for PSD, these techniques will not be covered in this review.

Table 3. Imaging variables (Computed Tomography and conventional Magnetic Resonance Imaging) relevant to study of poststroke dementia

A. Stroke related brain lesions	Remarks
Types	ischemic or hemorrhage
Sites	strategic sites
Relevance	symptomatic, silent, or old
Patterns	cortical, large subcortical, lacunar infarct or borderzone infarct
Laterality	dominant hemisphere
Multiplicity	single or multiple
Size	linear, planimetric, or volumetric
Extent	ventricular or subarachnoid extension for ICH
B. Whit matter changes	
Sites	periventricular and/or deep
Extent	visual grading of extent of WMC (thin cap or rim, halo, irregular, extending, punctate, patchy, or confluent), volumetric quantification*
C. Brain atrophy	
Cortical atrophy	sulci/fissures enlargement (visual, linear, planimetric, volumetric*), cortical gray matter global and regional (volumetric)*
Subcortical atrophy	ventricular enlargement (visual, linear, planimetric, volumetric)
General cerebral atrophy	ventricular brain ratio, ventricular cranial ratio (linear, planimetric, volumetric), total brain atrophy (volumetric)
Regional atrophy	hemispheric, frontal, parietal, temporal, hippocampal, corpus callosum (visual, planimetric* or volumetric*)
D. Others	
Perivascular space	FLAIR (hypointense) and T2-weighted MRI (hyperintense)*
Hippocampal sclerosis	coronal FLAIR and T2-weighted MRI (hyperintense)*

* Applicable mainly for MRI.

Computed Tomography

Routine CT is able to provide essential data relevant to PSD. Despite rapid advances in MRI techniques, CT will remain an important imaging modality in the study of PSD especially among developing countries given its low cost, wide availability, and simplicity in both technique and interpretation. Computed tomography can accurately detect surgical treatable dementias, such as subdural hemorrhage or hydrocephalus. Limitations of CT relevant to PSD include poor visualization of small infarcts and infratentorial lesions. Furthermore, assessment of temporal region, although is possible, [89] is usually difficult due to bone-hardening artifact and coronal images of CT, which has better visualization for medial temporal or hippocampal region, are difficult to obtain [90]. Note that with the rapid advances in CT techniques, some of these limitations may be overcome. For e.g., with the recent application of multidetector CT, smaller infarct may be visualized given its better spatial resolution.

In general, standard methods in the evaluation of stroke are also applicable for the evaluation of PSD. Contrast enhanced CT imaging has no specific role in the evaluation of PSD except in occasional case where cerebral malignancy or infection needs to be ruled out in stroke patient with dementia. Issues relating to the detection of acute cerebral infarctions by CT will not be discussed in this review.

1. Brain Lesions

Established cerebral infarcts appear as hypodense lesions on CT. Site (e.g. strategic sites), laterality (dominant versus non-dominant side) and pattern (e.g. lacunar, territorial cortical or large subcortical, borderzone) of the infarcts can be determined and involved vascular territories or mechanisms can then be implied. Differentiation between symptomatic, silent, or old infarct is mainly determined by correlation with clinical features. Lacunar infarct on CT is defined as a small, sharply demarcated round or oval hypodense area located along territory of small penetrating artery. Radiological limits for the size of lacunar infarct are commonly set between 3-20mm, which are larger than the pathological limits of 3-15mm. This is because surrounding edema of the infarct is also visualized by the neuoimaging. Although SVD is the commonest cause for lacunar infarct, subcortical lacunar infarct may also be associated with intra/extracranial large artery diseases and cardioembolism. Note that MCA atherosclerotic disease may not uncommonly induce subcortical lacunar infarcts due to blockage of the origin of a penetrating artery or microembolic phenomeon [32]. Hence, evaluation of intracranial large artery status by transcranial doppler ultrasound or CT / MR angiography is needed to assess the vascular etiology of lacunar infarct among ethnic groups (e.g. Asians, Blacks and Hispanics) where intracranial large artery disease is prevalent. This practice applies also to the use of MRI in the evaluation of lacunar infarcts. In evaluating ICH among those with PSD, apart from its site (e.g. strategic site, superficial or deep), laterality, and size, presence of ventricular/subarachnoid extension needs also to be assessed.

Linear measurement on the size of the ischemic or hemorrhagic lesion can be done manually and is usually represented by the greatest diameter of the lesion. Most of the CT workstation is able to quantify the surface area of the lesions at its greatest diameter. Volume of hematoma or infarcts can also be estimated via various formulas [41, 91] or by computerized automated methods [92]. The volume is the best measure in reflecting the size of the vascular lesion. Furthermore, various ratios of the infracted volumes over brain volume or brain volume minus ventricular volumes have been used in the study of PSD [93]. These ratios may be more relevant to cognitive impairment than the actual size of the lesions.

2. White Matter Changes

On CT, WMC are defined as patchy or diffuse symmetric areas of intermediate density, i.e. density between that of normal white matter and that of CSF, with ill-defined margins, located in the periventricular and/or the deep (centrum semiovale) white matter region (figure 2a). Different visual methods in rating its severity have been devised and have been used in cross-sectional studies [93-96]. Standard template has commonly been used as reference to grade severity. Qualitatively, the severity of WMC may vary from punctuate or fuzzy hypodensity at around the frontal or occipital horns to diffuse periventricular hypodensity with ill-defined margins extending into the deep white matter. The sensitivity of detecting WMC by CT is less than that by MRI in particular when WMC are small or are located at the parieto-occipital and infratentorial regions [94]. Inter-rater agreement of visual rating scale based on CT is generally less than that based on MRI [94, 96] Using CT based visual rating method to monitor WMC progression longitudinally for research purpose is generally not advisable as inter/intra-rater agreement will deem to be low. In principle, visual rating is highly rater dependable and is best used by a single rater for assessment of the same patient. Quantitative method in assessment of WMC by CT has not been applied as the margin between normal and abnormal white matter is poorly delineated by CT. Albeit the above disadvantages, CT findings of WMC may correlate more with clinical severity than that of conventional MRI due to higher specificity in detecting severe WMC by CT, whereas small area of hyperintense white matter signals detected by MRI may have no clinical relevance [97].

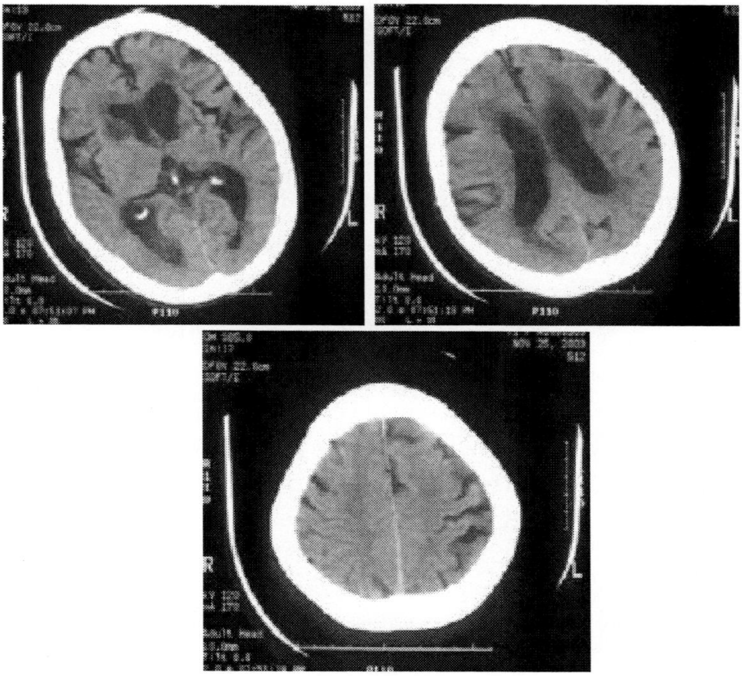

Figure 2. Subcortical vascular dementia. Figure 2a. Computed Tomography

Patient is a 73-year-old female with hypertension who presented with fall and acute confusion. Examination revealed small step gait with postural instability. Her MMSE was only 5/30. Initial CT (figure 2a) reveals multiple lacunar infarcts (more lacunar infarcts are present on other slices that are not shown here) and periventricular WMC extending into the centrum semiovale, with left side slightly more sever than the right side.

Geroldi et al had recently devised a CT-based method to rate the cerebral load of SVD [98]. Apart from severity of WMC, measures of lacunes were also incorporated into the scale. They attempted to construct the rating method with reference to clinical severity. In this rating method, they scored three types of SVD separately: (1) diffuse leukoaraiosis; (2) patchy hypodensity that exists within the leukoaraiosis and fuzzy hypodensity that exists outside the context of leukoaraiosis; and (3) lacunes. Weighting was then assigned to the score of each type of SVD based on its correlation with a scale that measures severity of extrapyramidal signs. A continuous score and an ordinal class with higher values indicating greater severity of SVD were derived accordingly by a formula and statistical methods respectively. The scoring system was found to have good inter/intra-rater reliability and correlation with vascular risk factors and physical impairment. Furthermore, patients diagnosed to have severe SVD based on conventional method were found more often to have higher class while those with AD were found more often to have lower class.

Note that radiological WMC are not only related to vascular etiology, and can be related to non-ischemic etiologies, e.g. multiple sclerosis, cerebral malignancy, or post radiation. Hence, acquiring patients' clinical background is important to interpret the nature of WMC during the evaluation of PSD.

3. Brain Atrophy

Method in assessing cerebral atrophy for PSD is similar to that in assessing for any dementia. Cortical, subcortical, general, or regional atrophy can be assessed qualitatively and quantitatively by CT using various methods [89, 90]. Widening of cortical sulci and fissures with relatively normal ventricular size reflect predominant cortical atrophy. Ventricular enlargement with relatively normal cortical sulci and fissures reflect predominant subcortical atrophy. Pattern of regional atrophy may also provide diagnostic clue for PSD. For example, severe predominant frontal lobe atrophy in PSD may suggest concurrent frontotemporal dementia. Ventricular enlargement of temporal horn and sylvian fissure enlargement may support concurrent AD in a demented patient with stroke and progressive prestroke cognitive impairment.

Various CT based visual rating scales on enlargement of sulci /fissures and ventricles are available [90, 93]. As in visual rating for WMC, standard template has been used as reference in grading cortical and subcortical atrophy. Linear measurements on the width of sulci /fissures and various regions of the ventricle may provide a more objective measure than visual scales. Linear measurements for the ventricle commonly include maximal distance between the lateral borders of the frontal horns, the sum of the shortest distances between the caudate and the anterior end of the septum pellucidum, the maximal width of the third ventricle, or the width of the bodies of the lateral ventricles at their waist. Apart from using the actual width of the ventricles, it is also common to divide the ventricular width by the width of the brain at the same level so as to take into account for the individual variation of the brain or head size. This gives the ventricular brain ratio

(VBR), [99] which is more of an index for general cerebral atrophy and is probably a more relevant index to cognitive impairment than the actual ventricular width [100]. Some had used the summation of various ventricular measures and divide it by the brain width to represent cerebral atrophy [101].

Planimetric measurement (cross sectional area) of the inter-hemispheric fissure, the brain surface area, or ventricular size, at a particular level can be determined quantitatively via the CT workstation [102, 103]. Finally, volumetric measurement for CSF space, intracranial or brain volume is also possible with various CT automated techniques [90, 92]. Area based VBR, volume based VBR or ventricular cranial ratio (VCR) can be calculated accordingly. Volumetric method is probably the best CT related measurement for assessing cerebral atrophy in terms of sensitivity, specificity, and reliability both for cross-sectional study or longitudinal study that evaluates progression of atrophy [90, 103] Although quantitative CT density has been used as a measurement for cerebral atrophy in the past, this method is now considered to be obsolete due to its invalidity in reflecting cerebral atrophy [90]. The limitation of CT in the assessment of atrophy of the medial temporal or hippocampal region has been discussed.

T1-, T2- and PD Weighted and FLAIR Magnetic Resonance Imaging

T1-, T2-, PD, and/or FLAIR that are based on spin echo (SE) techniques have become standard MRI protocols for the evaluation of ischemic PSD for many centers. Relative to CT, MRI in general has better differentiation between anatomical structures (e.g. gray matter, white matter and CSF), greater ease of imaging at different planes, e.g. coronal or sagittal, greater sensitivity in detecting infarcts, lacunar infarcts, or WMC, and better visualization of structures at the temporal region and posterior fossa given the absence of bone-hardening artifact and availability of coronal plan. Furthermore, different sequence that yields unique or complementary information can be obtained at a single scanning session, although a longer scanning time relative to CT is required. All these advantages of MRI make it the preferred imaging modality over CT in the evaluation of PSD.

1. Brain Lesions

Cerebral infarct is usually assessed by axial T1-weighted MRI and is seen as hypointense area. Principles of evaluation are similar to that used for CT. Site, laterality, pattern of infarct are determined. Coronal and/or sagittal section may help to better visualize the extent of infarct. As in CT, size of infarct on MRI can be represented by simple linear measurements of the widest diameter of the infarct. Areas and volumes of infarcts can be determined by various formulas or computerized program. Special caution is given to differentiate between lacunar infarct and perivascular space on MRI. Perivascular space is more visible on MRI than on CT given the better resolution of the former modality. Perivascular spaces are commonly located in the basal ganglia and centrum ovale. It may be punctate or linear. As with lacunar infarct, it is hypointense on T1-weighted imaging. In general, perivascular space is smaller than lacunar infarct. Pathological study with MRI correlation found that size of <3mm in diameter was highly predictive of perivascular space, [104] except around the anterior commissure, where perivascular spaces could be large. This criterion has been used in most studies for its differentiation. Methods of T1- and T2-weighted MRI in evaluation of ICH for PSD follow that of evaluation for stroke and will not be discussed in this review.

2. White Matter Changes

Relative to CT, MRI is superior in the detection of WMC. Traditionally, SE axial PD weighted and T2-weighted MRI imaging is used in the evaluation of WMC. In general, T1-weighted imaging is insensitive to detection of WMC (figure 2b) [105]. On PD weighted image, WMC are hyperintense but signal intensity is lower for CSF. Evaluation of periventricular WMC is hence best performed by PD weighted image because delineation between CSF and WMC is easier with PD weighted image, while it may sometimes be difficult with T2-weighted imaging as both appear bright on T2-weighted. Some center prefers using T2-weighted imaging over PD weighted in the evaluation of deep WMC as better contrast is exhibited between lesions and white matter with the former image [100] Note that recently fast SE has been increasingly used to acquire T2- and PD weighted imaging in view of time consideration. However, the CSF signal is brighter than that in a conventional SE, making differentiation between periventricular WMC and ventricle slightly more difficult. Hence, a “true” PD weighted image cannot be obtained with fast SE. A more recent technique in the evaluation of WMC is the use of FLAIR, where the CSF signal is attenuated by the use of a long inversion time that nullifies the signal of water (figure 2d). Periventricular WMC is hence easily differentiated from the ventricular CSF. Some studies have suggested that FLAIR is more sensitive and accurate in detection of periventricular and subcortical lesions than that of PD/T2-weighted imaging [94, 106] However, sensitivity of FLAIR is reduced at the posterior fossa and diencephalon region. It is as yet uncertain whether FLAIR can replace T2/PD weighted imaging in the evaluation of WMC.

Several descriptions on WMC related hyperintense signals on T2/PD-weighted or FLAIR have been used.

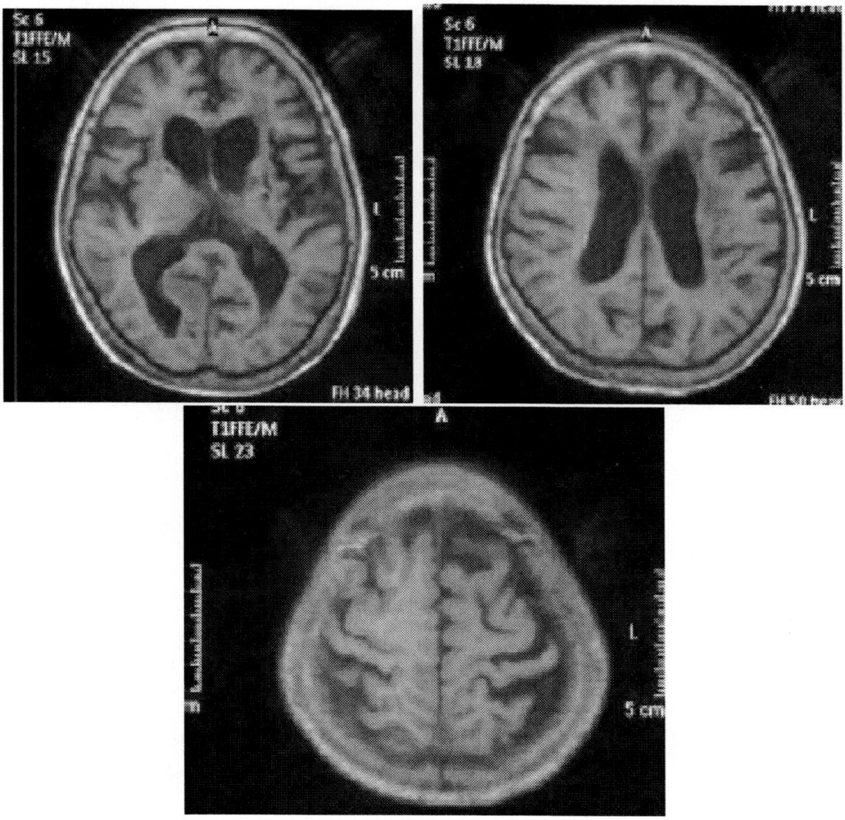

Figure 2b. T1-weighted

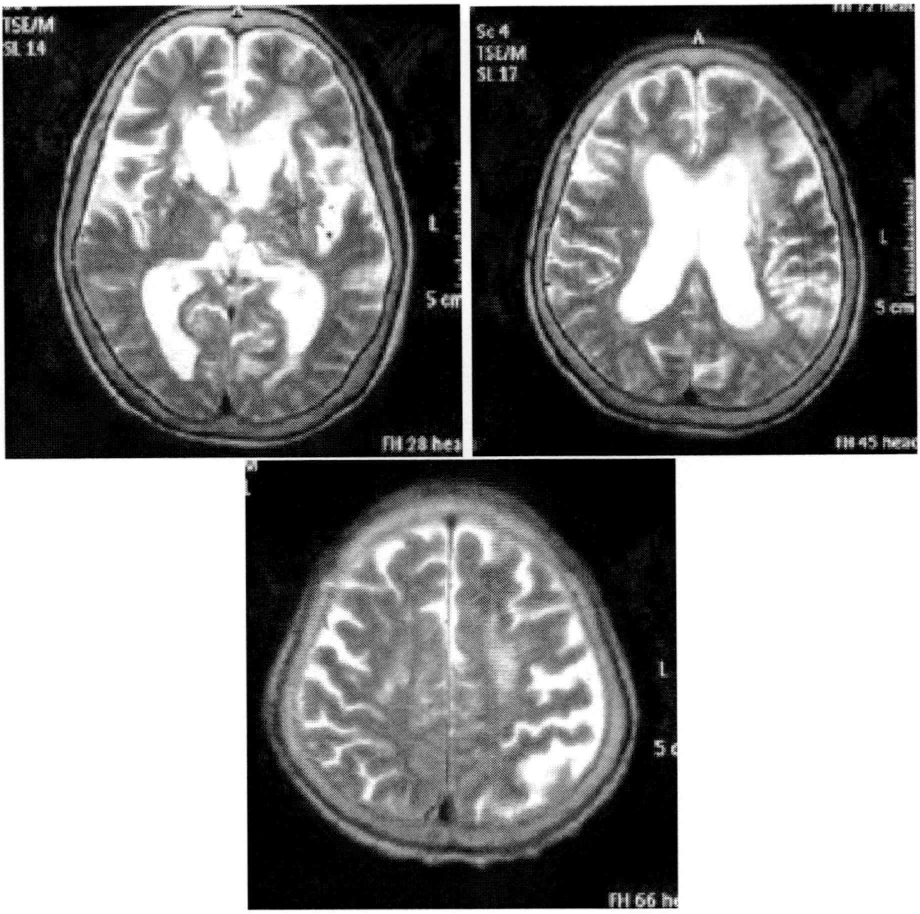

Figure 2c. T2-weighted

Hyperintensities around frontal and occipital horns are called "caps" and those around the lateral ventricles are described as "bands", "rims", "linings", "smooth halo", or "irregular" hyperintensities extending into the deep white matter. "Punctate", "focal", "patchy", and "confluent" have been used to describe extent of WMC, mostly at the deep white matter region.

On T2- weighted, PD weighted, or FLAIR imaging, WMC need to be distinguished from perviascular space. Perivascular space is hyperintense on T2-weighted, hypointense on FLAIR and relative hypointense or poorly visible on PD weighted, while WMC are hyperintense on all 3 imaging.

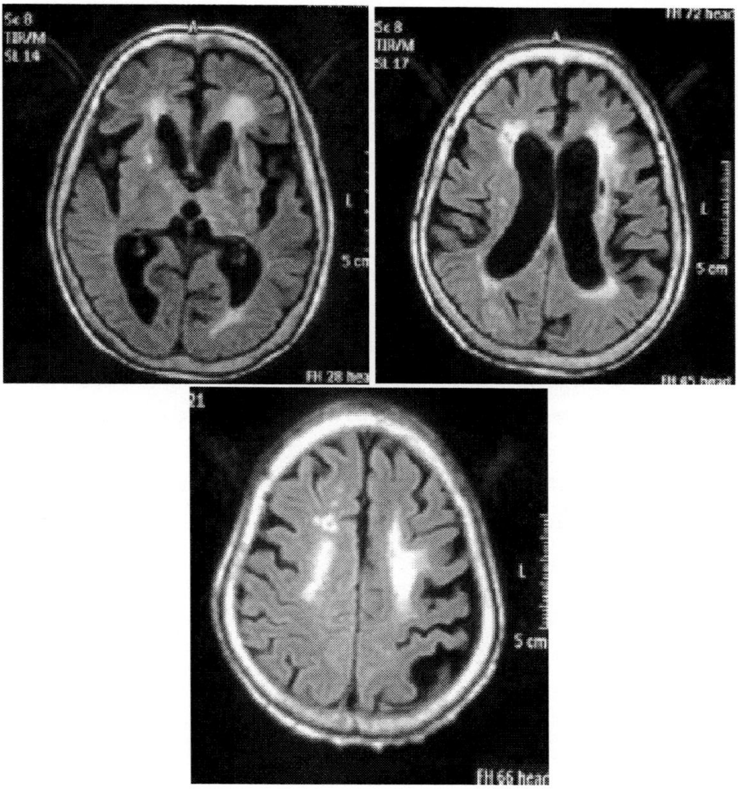

Figure 2d. FLAIR

MRI was performed 6 months after the event. T1-weighted (figure 2b) reveals multiple small hypointensities (lacunar infarcts). WMC are not well-visualized on T1weighted relative to T2-weighted (figure 2c) or FLAIR (figure 2d). Cortical atrophy of the frontal and parietal lobe (widening of Sylvian fissures and sulci, more prominent on the left) is present. Note that delineation between WMC and CSF is much more easier on FLAIR than that on T2-weighted.

Both visual and quantitative volumetric methods have been used to assess the severity of WMC on MRI. Multitude of MRI based visual rating scales are available [94, 96, 100, 107-110] and many of it have been summarized by Mantyla et al (see appendix) [111, 112]. The scales are in general more sophisticated than that based on CT given the better visualization of WMC by MRI over CT. Most of the scales rate periventricular and deep white matter region separately because pathology and relevance to cognition may vary with the location [67, 109]. Some scales only rate WMC at either periventricular or deep white matter region, while some scales give a combined rating of both regions

[111] Standard templates are commonly used for reference [100, 107]. The Wahlund's scale is applicable for both MRI and CT. [94]. In general, inter-rater agreement of the visual scales are acceptable and few of these scales, e.g. Manolio, Fazekas and Schmidt, and Sheltens and Wahlund, have good correlations with volumetric measures [107, 108, 110, 113]. However, comparative studies have demonstrated that different visual scales probably measure different aspects of WMC. This may explain the inconsistent findings regarding the frequency, extent, and clinical correlates of WMC [111]. Furthermore, for assessment of progression of WMC, studies found that visual scales showed little correlation with volumetrics and low inter-rater agreement [112, 114]. On this regard, a new "white matter lesion change scale" was recently proposed, showing better correlation with volumetric measure over time [112].

Volume of WMC can be determined quantitatively with MRI workstation using various automated methods [112-114]. Although volumetric measurement is probably the best method for both cross-sectional and longitudinal studies of WMC and its progression, the assessment time is longer and level of expertise is greater than that required with visual methods. Note that the volume of WMC can be represented as ratio over total brain or cranial volume too [115].

3. Brain Atrophy

Evaluation of brain atrophy with MRI provides more information with greater accuracy than that with CT because different planes and better visualization are possible with MRI. The usual protocol for atrophy measures includes axial and 3 dimensional coronal T1-weighted imaging. Global cortical atrophy can be assessed qualitatively by evaluation of size of sulci/fissures on axial T1-weighted imaging [107]. Qualitative regional cortical atrophy is also possible with frontal lobe (axial), [100] parietal lobe (coronal), [100] and medial temporal lobe (coronal) [100, 116]. Model templates for reference are commonly used [100, 107] Most of these visual methods have acceptable inter-rater agreement. Surface area of the corpus callosum can also be quantified via software program, yet a mid-sagittal plane is needed for its assessment [117]. Note that if the detection of hippocampal sclerosis is important, additional coronal T2-weighted or FLAIR image is also needed, which may demonstrate hippocampal hyperintensity in the presence of sclerosis. Recently, sophisticated quantitative volumetric method for assessing atrophy of cortical gray matter, both global and regional cortical atrophy, had been applied for study of PSD [115].

Apart from cortical atrophy, total brain, hemispheric and regional volumes including hippocampal volume can all be quantified by MRI techniques [115, 118, 119]. Longitudinal evaluation of change in cerebral atrophy can be done either serially, or more recently, by the registration plus subtraction technique [120].

Qualitative ratings of ventricular size using MRI have been used [107, 119]. Similar to CT, linear and planimetric measurements of the ventricle can be obtained via MRI and the data is usually represented as ratio over the respective brain measures to give the VBR [100, 121]. Absolute ventricular volume, volume based VBR or VCR can all be obtained by MRI and are relevant to study of dementia [115, 118].

PET, SPECT, and Xenon CT

While CT and above MRI sequences provide structural information, PET, SPECT, and xenon CT provide information on cerebral perfusion and/or metabolism, which reflect pathological process that is undetectable by structural imaging [36, 87, 92, 122-129]. These functional imaging techniques have been used in the study of PSD for over 2 decades.

1. Positron Emission Tomography

Positron emission tomography is the most sensitive and comprehensive, yet expensive functional imaging. It is able to determine quantitatively regional cerebral blood flow (CBF), oxygen metabolism ($CMRO_2$), oxygen extraction fraction (OEF), and /or glucose metabolism (CMRgl). ^{15}Oxygen steady state technique is commonly used for the determination of CBF, $CMRO_2$, and OEF, while flurodeoxyglucose tagged with ^{18}Fluroine (18 FDG) is the most commonly used isotope for determination of CMRgl in study of PSD. Strength of PET is that viability or metabolic reserve of brain tissue can be reflected by the pattern of metabolic parameters. For instance, increased OEF associated with reduced CBF and reduced/preserved $CMRO_2$ suggests misery perfusion and pending infarction.

2. Single Photon Emission Computed Tomography

Single photon emission computed tomography is less sensitive, yet less costly, and can provide regional cerebral semi-quantitative assessment on CBF. However, oxygen metabolism cannot be measured by SPECT. Furthermore, different to PET, it provides only ratios of perfusion at region of interest relative to another brain region and absolute CBF cannot be provided. $^{99}Tc^{m}$ labeled derivative of hexamethyl propylene amine oxime (MHPAO) has been the most frequently used tracer for study of PSD.

Since spatial resolution of PET and SPECT is poor, techniques in co-registering PET and SPECT images to CT or MRI have been used recently.

3. Xenon CT

Similar to SPECT, xenon CT only measures CBF. Although the intravenous ^{133}xenon method had been used to study PSD, [130] it has been replaced by stable xenon inhalation method. The later method permits differentiated measurement of cortical and subcortical structures. Although as in PET, absolute CBF can be determined, the potential side effects of inhaled xenon and its associated motion artifacts related to patient's movements, and the need of meticulous monitoring during the procedure, (e.g. electroencephalogram, electrocardiogram, blood pressure, arterial oxygen saturation, and/or end tidal carbon dioxide concentration), make use of xenon CT relatively limited.

4. Cerebral Vasoreactivity

Apart from cerebral perfusion and metabolism, cerebral vasoreactivity can also be assessed using above modalities. Use of inhaled carbon dioxide in the study of cerebral vasoreactivity has now been mostly replaced by acetazolamide due to patient's discomfort associated with the former agent. Intravenous injection of acetazolamide increases CBF by 30-40% in a patient with intact cerebral vasoreactivity. The inability to increase CBF following acetazolamide challenge suggests impaired cerebral vasoreactivity. The change in CBF from baseline can be determined by PET, SPECT, or xenon CT.

5. Functions and Findings of PET, SPECT, and Xenon CT in Poststroke Dementia

a. Pathophysiology of White Matter Changes

To date, studies in PSD using PET, SPECT, or xenon CT have served important functions in the study of PSD. First, it helps to elucidate the pathogenesis of WMC, which is an important substrate in PSD. An early study using ^{15}oxygen steady state PET technique among patients with subcortical VaD found that CBF was reduced at subcortical white matter region [127]. This further lends support to the ischemic origin for WMC and is consistent with the pathological findings and clinical association between WMC and vascular risk factors [131]. Although this same study failed to demonstrate an increase in OEF at any cerebral region, a later study by De Reuck et al had shown that OEF was significantly increased at all cerebral regions, including the white matter, among patients with lacunar dementia who had reduced CBF and $CMRO_2$. [87] This finding suggests that at least in some patients with subcortical VaD, chronic misery perfusion at the white matter region occurs. This provides insight and opportunity for potential therapeutic intervention. Furthermore, the same group had demonstrated that cerebral vasoreactivity was severely impaired at all cerebral regions using PET study with acetazolamide challenge [132]. Hence, apart from narrowed small arteries, ischemia may be further compounded by impaired regulatory reserve, which is particularly detrimental to the white matter in the presence of postural hypotensive change, low output cardiac failure, or aggressive anti-hypertensive treatment. Note that although, reduced subcortical CBF and CMRgl among patients with severe SVD have been demonstrated by most studies, Sabri et al failed to demonstrate such an association [126].

b. Mechanisms of Poststroke Dementia

More importantly, the various functional imaging have helped to elucidate the mechanisms of dementia in PSD, especially for PSD associated with subcortical brain lesions. Studies have consistently demonstrated that subcortical lesions, either single strategic lesion or diffuse ischemic lesions, are associated with cortical hypometabolism and/or hypoperfusion despite absence of structural cortical lesions, [36, 87, 123, 124, 127] and that these metabolic or perfusional abnormalities correlate with cognitive performances [123, 124, 129] and even predict cognitive progression [125]. These findings support that disconnection of subcortical white matter fiber tracts or specific circuits may be responsible for the PSD. An earlier study found that the correlation between hypoperfusion and cognitive impairment was particularly strong among stroke patients (mostly lacunar stroke) with mild dementia (mini-mental state examination [MMSE] of >15), whereas this correlation was weak among severely demented patients with larger infarcts [92]. In the later group, infarct volume was found to be more relevant than hypoperfusion in determining cognitive performance. Though it must be emphasized that in another study, the hypoperfusion was found to extend beyond the infracted areas among those with large infarct, and hence hypoperfusion may also affect cognitive performances independent of volume of infarct even among those with large infarct [87].

c. Differentiation between Etiologies of Dementia

Given that unique pattern of hypometabolism and hypoperfusion exists in AD and subcortical ischemic lesions, functional imaging may help to delineate the contribution of each disease in accounting for the dementia poststroke. This is particularly useful in case where such delineation is difficult, e.g. progressive cognitive decline occurs after a small lacunar stroke. Using 18 FDG PET, Reed et al demonstrated that among cognitive impaired stroke patient with subcortical lacunar infarct, memory loss correlated with prefrontal lobe hypometabolism, whereas in AD (but not in subcortical lacunar infarct), memory correlated with hippocampal and temporal lobe hypometabolism [129].

In general, irrespective of subtypes of VaD, pattern of hypometabolism will be more focal, patchy and variable affecting cortical and subcortical areas, compared with typical hypometabolism affecting the parietotemporal association areas seen in AD.

d. Monitoring Effects of Therapy

Positron emission tomography has also been utilized in monitoring the effect of drug therapy. An early study demonstrated that CBF as measured by PET could be increased by certain drug (e.g. propentofylline) and this improvement correlated with clinical stabilization [133]. A recent study also evaluated the effect of cholinesterase inhibitor on regional CBF among patients with poststroke VaD [134]. This study shown that the drug increased CBF, which was more significant in the frontal region among the treated patients, and suggested that cholinesterase inhibitor might regulate CBF and such effects were more pronounced in the more affected brain region.

In summary, the value of PET, SPECT, and xenon CT in study of PSD cannot be underestimated. Yet, its cost, complexity and/or the potential problems associated with the availability and use of radioactive tracer, have limited its use mainly for research purpose.

I. Imaging Determinants for Ischemic Poststroke Dementia

Poststroke Dementia at Three Months

Few recent large hospital-based prospective studies have yielded various imaging determinants for PSD based on multivariate regression analyses. Imaging determinants based on studies that evaluated PSD (i.e. including those with prestroke dementia and prior stroke) 3 months poststroke include [17, 48, 50, 70] volume of infarcts in any superior middle cerebral artery, [17] any [48, 70] or number (mostly lacunar infarcts) of left sided infarcts, [17] lacunar infarct, [70] extent of WMC, [17] and medial temporal lobe atrophy [17]. Note that for studies demonstrating the relevance of left sided infarcts, patients with severe aphasia were excluded, [17, 48, 70] hence suggesting that left sided lesions can also be associated with global cognitive impairment. Findings of our recent study are similar to previous studies in that extent of WMC, MCA territorial infarct, and cerebral atrophy measure were found to predict PSD. [50]. It appears that large infarct along MCA territory, lacunar infarcts and its frequency, left sided laterality, extent of WMC, general cerebral atrophy, and medial temporal lobe atrophy all correlate with PSD in general.

Two of the above studies had performed sub-analyses upon those with new onset dementia at 3 months poststroke [17, 50]. Number of relevant imaging features decreased after excluding those with prestroke dementia. Volume of left anterior corona radiata infarct, which is probably a strategic site, became the only determinant in one study [17]. Extent of WMC remained a strong determinant in our study [50]. In general, influence of general cerebral atrophy or medial temporal lobe atrophy decrease when patients with prestroke dementia were excluded. A large proportion of these excluded patients might probably have underlying AD. While vascular factors, such as volume of left sided anterior corona radiata infarct or extent of WMC, play more important role in new onset dementia at 3 months poststroke.

Two recent studies evaluated dementia at 3 months poststroke among those with first stroke (excluding prior stroke). [73, 135]. Volume of left sided anterior corona radiata infarct, [135] large MCA territory infarction, [73] frontal lobe lesion, [73] extent of WMC, [135] and medial temporal lobe atrophy [135] were found to predict dementia. These determinants are similar to studies including patients with any dementia in that the relevance of left sided anterior infarct, extent of WMC, and medial temporal lobe atrophy were demonstrated.

Delayed Poststroke Dementia

Few studies also evaluated the imaging determinants of delayed PSD at mean follow up of 3-4 years [18, 19, 136]. These studies had excluded those with prestroke dementia. Baseline imaging features that were found to predict delayed PSD were extent of WMC, [19, 136] silent infarct, [19] multiple ischemic lesions (mostly lacunar infarcts), [18] and cortical atrophy [18]. Only one of these studies evaluated the influence of medial temporal lobe atrophy on delayed PSD, but failed to demonstrate such an association [136]. An interesting finding noted by 2 separate studies is that etiology for incident dementia shifted from Alzheimer' type in the first year to VaD type in later years [18, 19]. This suggests that vascular lesions may unmask an underlying asymptomatic AD early on poststroke, while the cerebral vascular load predisposes development of VaD in later years.

The above findings are derived from hospital-based studies, which may not represent the general population. To our knowledge, community study that investigates imaging determinants for PSD is lacking. Yet, the consistent pattern observed in the above hospital-based studies increases the validity of their findings.

Lacunar Infarct, Cognitive Impairment and Dementia

Imaging determinants for dementia or cognitive impairment among stroke associated with lacunar infarct have been particularly studied given that SVD is probably the most prevalent form of VaD [14, 86, 95, 115, 126, 137-142]. Although some of these studies investigated imaging correlates among patients with varying severity levels of cognitive impairment, from normal, mild to severe cognitive impairment (dementia) [86, 140-142] and some studies included random sample of patients with lacunar infarcts who might or might not suffer from overt stroke, [86, 115, 141] these studies will also be included given its potential relevance of PSD among lacunar stroke.

Miyao et al found that among those with WMC, more patients developed dementia over a period of 2 years poststroke than those without it [139]. However, influence of cerebral atrophy was not assessed in that study. In another study by Loeb et al, cerebral atrophy, rather than WMC, was found to predict dementia 4 years after lacunar stroke [95]. We demonstrated that WMC correlated with performance in executive tests and not in MMSE, [138] yet its severity did not predict dementia at 3 months after lacunar stroke [14]. Furthermore, when atrophy measures and site of lacunar infarct were added into the analyses, significance of WMC disappeared, whereas left frontal lobe atrophy and presence of thalamic lacune became significant predictors of cognitive performances [142]. Studies by Fein et al and Mungas et al demonstrated that atrophy of cortical gray matter and hippocampus, rather than WMC and lacunar infarcts, was the strongest determinant for dementia and cognitive performances in those with lacunar infarcts; and that WMC mainly correlated with performance on executive measure [115, 137]. Furthermore, baseline cortical atrophy, rather than ischemic measures (WMC and lacunes), was found to predict cognitive decline over a period of 3 years [86]. Sabri et al also noted similar findings in that cerebral atrophy, rather than ischemic measures, predicted cognitive impairment in those with lacunar stroke [126]. The importance of cerebral or cortical atrophy is consistent with findings based on functional imaging studies in that cortical, cerebral or frontal lobe hypometabolism and hypoperfusion were found to correlate with cognitive performances [123, 124, 129].

Yamauchi et al particularly investigated influence of corpus callosal atrophy in patients with lacunar infarcts and WMC and noted that the former predicted performance in MMSE while the later predicted performance in executive task [117].

Based on the above findings, it appears that in patients with lacunar stroke, various measures of brain atrophy, including cerebral, cortical, or regional (frontal lobe, hippocampus, corpus callosum) atrophy, are stronger determinants for cognitive performances and dementia over WMC. White matter changes affect mainly executive function and its association with severe cognitive impairment or dementia is less definitive.

The mechanisms for brain atrophy in patients with lacunar stroke deserve further remarks as one may argue that the atrophy is due to concurrent AD, which may also account for the cognitive impairment. Yet, pattern of cortical atrophy based on structural and functional studies in those with lacunar stroke is different to those with AD [115, 129]. Hypotheses for this atrophy include secondary axonal and trans-synaptic degeneration following primary subcortical ischemic injury and subclinical microinfarcts not visible by neuroimaging. In fact, cortical and callosal atrophy were found to correlate with extent of ischemic WMC [115, 140] The mechanisms for hippocampal atrophy in patients with lacunar infarcts are probably more variable, which include concurrent AD, hippocampal sclerosis, secondary degeneration, subclinical ischemia, or other unknown pathogenic processes [115].

White Matter Changes and Cognitive Impairment

As mentioned above, WMC are important imaging determinant for PSD and for executive dysfunction. There are certain factors that need also to be considered in the evaluation of the relationship between WMC and cognitive impairment. First, the relationship between WMC and cognitive impairment may not be linear and that a certain severity threshold of WMC may need to be exceeded before significant cognitive decline is induced. Our recent study suggested that the correlation of WMC with executive dysfunction might only be significant for marked WMC [138]. Second, cognitive impact of WMC may vary with its location. Periventricular lesion may induce greater cognitive impairment than deep WMC [109]. Hence studies that evaluated total WMC might dilute the cognitive influence of region specific WMC. Third, cognitive effect of WMC was recently shown to vary with educational level [143]. Those who are highly educated may have normal cognition despite having severe WMC. Fourth, the conventional imaging techniques may be either too sensitive or non- specific in detecting actual ischemic white matter lesions, given that radiological WMC may represent varying pathological changes as discussed previously [67]. Last, traditional criteria were used in many studies to define dementia. These criteria place less emphasis on executive dysfunction. Furthermore, psychometric batteries used in studies might not be comprehensive for the assessment of executive dysfunction. Hence, the impact of WMC might be underestimated.

Strategic Infarct Dementia (Figure 1)

Over the years, small case series reported the occurrence of new onset persistent dementia after a single stroke involving certain strategic areas in the absence of other relevant brain lesions such as severe WMC or atrophy that might account for the dementia. These areas include thalamus, angular gyrus, genu of the left internal capsule, anterior corpus callosum, inferior medial temporal lobe, hippocampus, frontal lobe, and caudate nucleus [34-37]. Strategic single infarct dementia accounts less than 10% of VaD [35]. Although, exact data regarding concomitant WMC and brain atrophy are lacking in most of these case series, most authorities accept this concept.

Cerebellar Infarct and Cognitive Impairment

Although risk of PSD after cerebellar infarct is lower relative to hemispheric infarct and association between cerebellar stroke and dementia has not been emphasized, [48] case series on infratentorial infarct (mostly cerebellar infarct) based on MRI demonstrated that executive function and visuospatial skills were impaired in cerebellar infarct, furthermore, global intelligence decline or dementia might result if large areas are involved. This study suggested the existence of certain cerebrocerebellar circuits that may be relevant to both motor and cognitive functions [144].

CADASIL and Imaging Features

CADASIL is an inhereditary disease affecting small arteries secondary to mutations within the *Notch3* gene and is associated with young stroke, dementia, migraine-like headaches, seizures, and other behavioral and motor features similar to that of subcortical VaD. Although in general it is uncommon, it is the commonest form of genetic form of PSD. Imaging features are similar to that of subcortical VaD, in that diffuse WMC and multiple lacunar infarcts are present. Yet certain imaging features help to differentiate between the two. Auer et al demonstrated with MRI (T2-weighted and FLAIR) that CADASIL patients had more extensive bilateral temporal, temporopolar and superior frontal WMC and bilateral signal reductions within the dentate nucleus, deep cerebellar white matter, crus cerebri, and thalamus [145]. Imaging determinants of cognitive impairment in CADASIL include quantitative volume of WMC on MRI [146] and cerebral hypometabolism on PET [147].

Perivascular Space and Cognitive Impairment

Although perivascular space is associated with ageing, SVD, and cerebral atrophy, it is considered to be clinically silent and is not routinely evaluated in PSD. However, dilated and multiple perivascular space (état criblé) may rarely associate with dementia in the absence of other pathologies [148]. Hence, perviascular space must be noted during imaging study if it is particularly severe.

Imaging Criteria for Poststroke Vascular Dementia (Table 4)

As mentioned earlier in this review, several clinical diagnostic criteria have been proposed to aid in diagnosing VaD and its subtypes [16, 20, 23, 26]. Imaging criteria have been incorporated into few of these criteria as objective evidence for the presence and relevance of CVD [16, 23, 26]. Most of the imaging criteria were developed more than 10 years ago, which were based on studies and case series on PSD that preceded the development of the criteria. Imaging criteria differ from imaging determinants of PSD. The former helps to determine the vascular contribution in PSD while the later predicts whether dementia will develop poststroke. Among the various diagnostic criteria for VaD, the NINDS-AIREN has the most specific imaging criteria and this set of imaging criteria will be discussed first.

NINDS-AIREN Imaging Criteria (Tables 1b and 4a)

The NINDS-AIREN task force emphasized that probable VaD could not be made without imaging abnormality in vivo irrespective of any stroke like clinical or physical features [16]. Although recognizing there are no pathognomonic brain CT or MRI images for VaD, they proposed a list of radiological findings describing both "topography" and "severity" of the lesions that favor diagnosis of

VaD. The strength of the NINDS-AIREN criteria is its high specificity in diagnosing VaD, [149] hence it has been the most widely used criteria in clinical studies. However, its sensitivity is low [25]. Patients with genuine poststroke VaD may be excluded from the study and hence findings from studies may not be generalized (figure 3). Furthermore, van Straaten et al found that the inter-rater agreement on its imaging criteria was low [150]. Part of the reason they noted was that specifications on certain items are lacking in the original criteria. For examples, the original criteria did not specify the exact number that is needed to be qualified as "multiple" lacunar infarcts, or the methods in approximating 25% of the total white matter for defining extensive WMC. In the same study, they discussed areas of uncertainties and then they operationalized it by adding relevant specifications, yet without changing the key contents of the criteria (table 4a). Inter-rater agreement improved slightly afterwards, mainly among the experienced raters.

Note that although the NINDS-AIREN criteria may help to determine the vascular contribution in a stroke patient with dementia, it may not predict the development of dementia poststroke. Ballard et al recently shown that among 125 consecutive stroke patients without prestroke dementia, no significant differences were noted between patients with and without PSD on any criteria of the imaging parameters within the NINDS-AIREN criteria [151]. The only different imaging feature was that hippocampal atrophy was more severe in those with PSD over those without PSD. Note that the average age of that cohort was about 10 years older than that of other studies on PSD. Hence, the predictive power of the NINDS-AIREN criteria for development of dementia is low, which may be particularly true among older stroke patients where hippocampal atrophy may have greater cognitive influence.

In summary, we propose that modification is needed for the NINDS-AIREN imaging criteria to improve its sensitivity and the criteria should preferably be operationalized to improve its inter-rater agreement.

Imaging Criteria for Subcortical VaD (Table 4b)

As mentioned earlier, research criteria have been recently proposed for diagnosis of subcortical VaD [26]. Imaging criteria based on both CT and MRI have been incorporated into this set of criteria. The extent of WMC and number of lacunar infarcts has been specified. Similar to NINDS-AIREN imaging criteria, it serves not to predict dementia among stroke patients. Yet, applying this set of imaging criteria among stroke patients, significantly more demented patients were noted among those with MRI fulfilling the criteria (40.7%) than patients with MRI not fulfilling the criteria (28.7%). Furthermore, those with MRI-defined severe SVD had less severe stroke but greater functional dependence, more depression, and apraxic gait disorders than those with other stroke subtypes. Albeit the imaging criteria have not been subjected to pathological validation study, it appears that the criteria are able to select a unique group of patients.

ADDTC (Table 1c)

Overall, the ADDTC is more conservative in linking particular type and pattern of vascular related brain lesions with dementia [23]. Hence, the imaging criteria are less stringent and specific than the NINDS-AIREN. To qualify a demented case as probable ischemic VaD, the criteria only require evidence of at least one infarct outside the cerebellum by CT or T1-weighted MRI. Presence of multiple infarcts in brain regions known to affect cognition is considered as supportive of probable VaD. However, the exact number and sites of brain infarcts have not been specified. Although periventricular and deep WMC on T2-weighted MRI that are excessive for age are mentioned to be potentially related with VaD, the criteria suggest that further research is needed before defining its relevance. Overall, given the less restrictions, the ADDTC has higher sensitivity than the NINDS-AIREN criteria, yet its specificity is lower [24, 25].

Imaging Criteria by Pullicino et al. [84] (Table 4c)

Pullicino et al proposed imaging criteria that could be used to predict the certainty of VaD [84]. The design of the criteria was based on the assumption that severity of vascular related brain damage correlates with the proportion of vascular component that contributes to the dementia syndrome and to the severity of dementia. The severity of vascular brain damage is reflected by the number and volume of infarcts (estimation by formula), severity of WMC (visual rating), and atrophy index[101] based on CT. Certainty of VaD is divided into four grades. Using these criteria with NINDS-AIREN as the reference, 78% of patients with grade 3 severity were classified correctly as having probable VaD, while 7% of those with grade 0 severity were classified correctly as no VaD. Intermediate grades (1 or 2) probably reflected mixed dementia. Furthermore, imaging grading was found to correlate with severity of cognitive impairment among those with CVD. The limitations of these criteria however are that small strategic infarcts may be misclassified as having no VaD and that severe WMC may not always associate with severe cognitive impairment. Although further modification and validation against pathology study is needed before its clinical application, this study highlights the potential utility of incorporating qualitative and/or quantitative assessment of multiple measures of vascular related brain lesions into the imaging criteria for VaD.

Other Imaging Criteria

The lack of imaging criteria in HIS probably affects is sensitivity in detecting vascular components. Loeb and Gandolfo proposed a simplified version of HIS that incorporated imaging features 2 decades ago [152]. They assigned score of 2 and 3 for those with isolated and multiple CT hypodensity respectively. However, its application in recent studies is scarce. In DSM IV [21] and ICD-10 [22] criteria for VaD, need of imaging evidence for CVD is only optional.

Table 4. Imaging criteria for poststroke dementia

4a. Operationalized imaging criteria of NINDS-AIREN criteria

Topography
- Large-vessel stroke – Large-vessel stroke is an infarction defined as a parenchymal defect in an arterial territory involving the cortical gray matter
- ACA – only bilateral ACA infarcts are sufficient to meet the NINDS-AIREN criteria
- PCA – infarcts in the PCA territory can be included only when they involve the following regions: Paramedian thalamic infarction: the infarct includes the cortical gray matter of the temporal/occipital lobe and extends into the paramedian part (defined as extending to the third ventricle) of the thalamus; the extension may be limited to the gliotic rim of the infarct that surrounds the parenchymal defect
- Inferior medical temporal lobe lesions

Association areas – an MCA infarction needs to involve the following regions:
- Parietotemporal: the infarct involves both the parietal and temporal lobe (e.g, angular gyrus)
- Temporo-occipital: the infarct involves both the temporal and occipital lobe

Table 4a. Continued

Watershed carotid territories – a watershed infarction is defined as an infarct in the watershed area between the MCA and PCA or the MCA and ACA in the following regions:

- Superior frontal region
- Parietal region

Small-vessel disease

Ischemic pathology resulting from occlusion of small perforating arteries may manifest itself as lacunes or white matter lesions. Lacune is defined as a lesion with CSF-like intensity on all sequences on MRI (water density on CT) surrounded by white matter or subcortical gray matter > 2mm. Care should be taken not to include Virchow-Robin spaces, which typically occur at the vertex and around the anterior commisure near the substantia perforata.

Ischemic white matter lesions are defined as circumscribed abnormalities with high signal on T2-weighted images not following CSF signal (mildly hypodense compared with surrounding tissue on CT) with a minimum diameter of 2 mm.

Multiple basal ganglia and frontal white matter lacunes – criteria are met when at lest 2 lacunes in the basal ganglia region (including thalamus and internal capsule) and at lest 2 lacunes in the frontal white matter are present.

Extensive periventricular white matter lesions in the white matter abutting the ventricles and extending irregularly into the deep white matter, or deep/subcortical white matter lesions. Smooth caps and bands by themselves are not sufficient. Gliotic areas surrounding large-vessel strokes should not be included here.

Bilateral thalamic lesion – to meet the criteria, at least 1 lesion in each thalamus should be present.

Severity

Large-vessel disease of the dominant hemisphere – if there is a large-vessel infarct as defined above, to meet the criteria it has to be in the dominant hemisphere. In the absence of clinical information, the left hemisphere is considered dominant.

Bilateral large-vessel hemispheric strokes – 1 of the infarcts should involve an area listed under topography but is in the nondominant hemisphere, while the infarct in the dominant hemisphere does not meet the topography criteria.

Leukoencephalopathy involving at lest ¼ of the total white matter when they are confluent (grade 3 in the ARWMC scale) in at least 2 regions of the ARWMC scale and beginning confluent (grade 2 in the ARWMC scale) in 2 other regions. A lesion is considered confluent when >20 mm or consists of ≥2 smaller lesions fused by more than connecting bridges.

Fulfillment of radiological criteria for probable VaD

Large-vessel disease – both the topography and severity criteria should be met (a lesion must be scored in at least 1 subsection of both topography and severity).

Small-vessel disease – for white matter lesions, both the topography and severity criteria should be met (a lesion must be scored in at least 1 subsection of both topography and severity); for multiple lacunes and bilateral thalamic lesions, only the topography criterion is sufficient.

ACA indicates anterior cerebral artery; PCA, posterior cerebral artery; MCA, middle cerebral artery; CSF, cerebrospinal fluid; and ARWMC, age-related white matter changes.

4b. Imaging criteria for subcortical VaD

A. Computed tomography

Extending periventricular and deep white matter lesions: patchy or diffuse symmetrical areas of low attenuation (intermediate density between that of normal white matter and that of intraventricular cerebrospinal fluid) with ill defined margins extending to the centrum semiovale, and at least one lacunar infarct.

AND

Absence of cortical and/or cortico-subcortical non-lacunar territorial infarcts and watershed infarcts, haemorrhages indicating large vessel disease, signs of normal pressure hydrocephalus, and specific causes of white matter lesions (e.g. multiple sclerosis, sarcoidosis, brain irradiation).

B. Magnetic resonance imaging

- To include predominantly "white matter cases"; extending periventricular and deep white matter lesions: extending caps (>10 mm as measured parallel to ventricle) or irregular halo (>10 mm broad, irregular margins and extending into deep white matter) and diffusely confluent hyperintensities (>25 mm, irregular shape) or extensive white matter change (diffuse hyperintensity without focal lesions), and lacune(s) in the deep gray matter.

OR

- To include predominantly "lacunar cases": multiple lacunes (e.g. >5) in the deep gray matter and at least moderate white matter lesions: extending caps or irregular halo or diffusely confluent hyperintensities or extensive white matter changes.

AND

- Absence of cortical and/or cortico-subcortical non-lacunar territorial infarcts and watershed infarcts, haemorrhages, signs of normal pressure hydrocephalus, and specific causes of white matter lesions (e.g. multiple sclerosis, sarcoidosis, brain irradiation).

4c. Pullicino's imaging criteria

Grade	Description	Criteria†
0	VaD absent	No infarcts; WMS, <3; VI, any dimension
1	VaD unlikely	Single infarct; VOL, <100 mL; Vl, any dimension
2	VaD possible	Multiple infarcts; VOL, <100 mL; Vl, ≥60
		Infarct(s); VOL, ≥100 mL; Vl, <60
		WMS, 3; Vl, ≥60
		WMS, 4; Vl, <60
3	VaD probable	Infarct(s); VOL, ≥100 mL; Vl, ≥60
		WMS, 4; Vl, ≥60

VOL, infarct volume; Vl, ventricular index; and WMS, white matter scale. †Each line gives a different allowable combination for that particular grade.

J. Recent Imaging Applications in PSD

Recent imaging applications in PSD include using either advanced techniques or techniques that have been well established in other areas but have recently been applied also in PSD. Most of these techniques revolve around MRI.

Diffusion Weighted Imaging

In brief, DWI measures the self-diffusion of water. In conventional MRI, diffusion effects are negligible. Application of a strong magnetic field gradient to an imaging pulse sequence allows diffusion sensitivity to be measurable. Strength and deviation of the gradient pulse determine the degree of diffusion weighting, which is expressed by the "b-value" of the sequence in s/mm^2. Higher b values of up to 1000 s/mm^2 are required to obtain a good contrast. Diffusion gradients are applied in at least 3 orthogonal directions. These images are usually combined to give the "trace" image, which represents the geometric mean of the individual images. In regions of acute cerebral infarcts where diffusion of water is restricted, the lesions appear hyperintense on DWI (figure 2f). Apparent diffusion coefficients (ADC) map can also be calculated from acquisitions with different b-values. In infarcted tissues with restricted water mobility, ADC maps appear dark and the regional ADC value is lower (figure 2f). Its superiority in detection of acute cerebral infarct over that of conventional MRI has been well established. In PSD, DWI may help to determine the site of acute infarct accurately during the first few days poststroke and to differentiate between acute and old/silent infarcts with reference to conventional MRI.

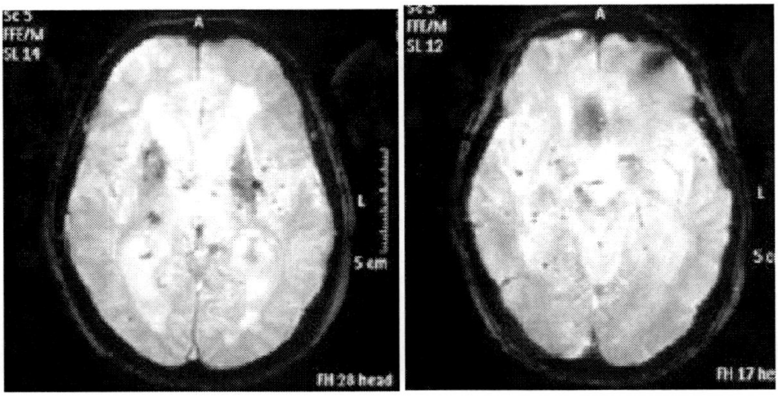

Figure 2e. T2*GE

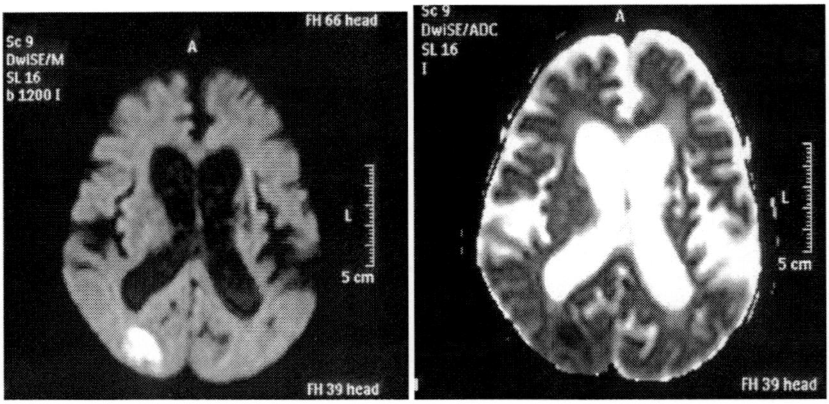

Figure 2f. DWI (left) and ADC map (right)

T2* GE MRI (figure 2e) of the same patient showing scattered small round hyointensities of varying size, which represent microbleeds. DWI at b=1200 s/mm^2 (figure 2f, left) reveals a "subclinical" acute infarct (hyperintense) at right occipital area that corresponds with hypointensity on the ADC maps (figure 2f, right). The patient was clinically stable at time of MRI. Note that the size of the acute infarct is relatively large and is located near the surface. MRA (not shown here) revealed severe stenosis of the posterior cerebral artery. This patient had mixed large and small artery disease.

Recent studies have suggested the potential of using DWI in assessing disease activity in those with SVD, subcortical VaD, or CADASIL [153, 154]. These studies demonstrated the occasional presence of "subclinical" recent lacunar infarcts based on DWI among patients with lacunar infarcts (8%), subcortical VaD (20%), and CADASIL (10.5%) who had no recent overt stroke event. The authors suggested that that presence of recent subclinical infarcts might reflect active disease. Further study is needed to assess whether it predicts rate of cognitive decline and whether it can be used as a surrogate marker in clinical trials.

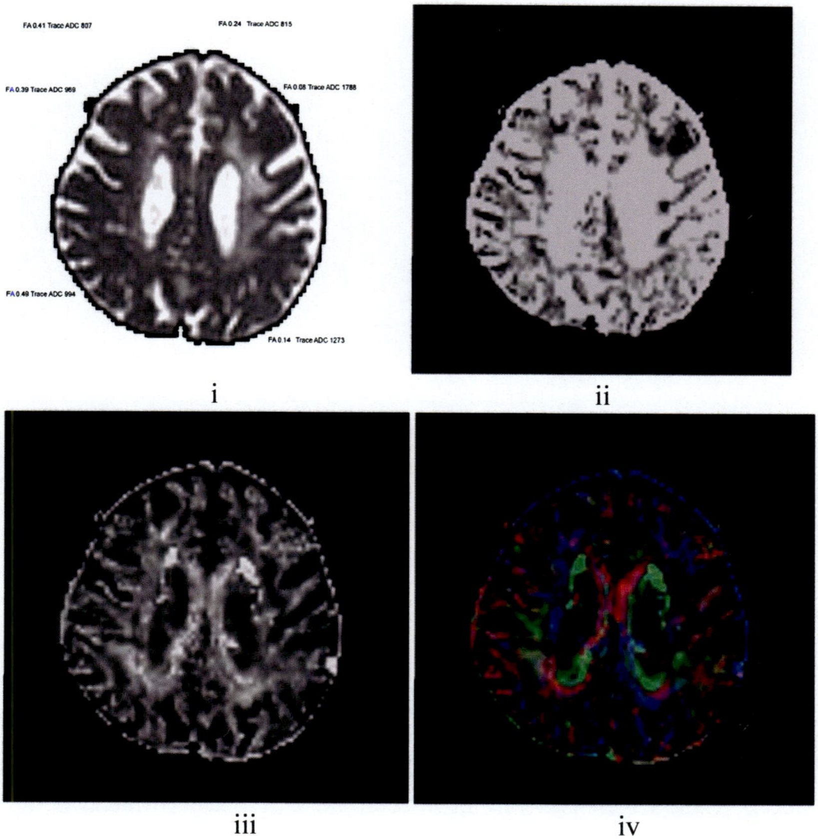

Figure 2g. i. B0; ii. Diffusion trace; iii. FA; iv. Color FA

Regions of interest were placed at normal appearing white matter on right (yellow cross) and left side (red cross) (figure 2g I, B0 image). The diffusion trace (figure 2g ii, x10^9 s/mm^2) at the left red cross (0.615) was slightly higher than that on the right yellow cross (0.607), while the FA (figure 2g iii) at the left (0.24) was lower than that at the right (0.41). This is suggestive of more severe damage of white matter fibre on the left than on the right side. The trace was higher and FA was lower at regions of WMC than that at normal appearing white matter (values not shown). In the color FA (figure 2g iv), each color represents fibres running at different direction (green=anterior-posterior, blue=caudal-cephalic, red=right-left).

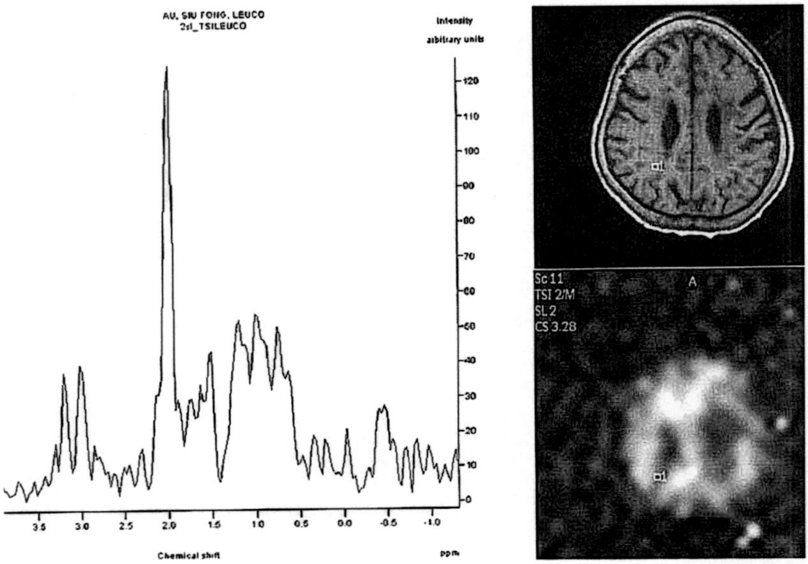

Figure 2h. ^{1}H MRS

A single voxel MRS study at right posterior white matter region. The spectrum with various peaks of the metabolites is shown on the right. MRS study at different regions may help to elucidate the mechanism of dementia in subcortical VaD and differentiate it from other types of dementing illnesses (see text).

Diffusion Tensor Imaging

Perhaps more important to the study of PSD is the recently developed MR technique of DTI, which is a further development of DWI. In the CSF or gray matter, diffusion is "isotropic", i.e. water can diffuse equally and easily in each direction, while in white matter myelinated fiber, diffusion is restricted in a sense that water molecules move preferentially along a fiber rather than perpendicular to it. This type of diffusion behavior is called "anisotropic" diffusion and the ADC at a point varies according to the direction in which it is measured. Determination of the complete diffusion information requires DWI with at least six diffusion-encoding gradient directions and the diffusion properties are described mathematically by a tensor. A tensor is a matrix of values; each corresponds to a gradient orientation and a cell orientation. The diffusion tensor MRI can provide information about the integrity of white matter tracts by estimation of the diffusion trace (i.e. averaged ADC) and the directionality. The later is commonly expressed as the fractional anisotropy (FA).

As mentioned before that WMC as shown on conventional MRI may represent heterogeneous pathologies, DTI can now provide a more specific measure for ischemic pathological WMC, i.e. loss of axons and myelins and gliosis. Jones et al found that in region of WMC, diffusion trace was elevated and FA was reduced, and that the elevation of trace was less than that found in large mature infarcts.[155] These changes are consistent with axonal loss and gliosis as loss of axons will result in increased diffusion, but the extent of this increase is probably limited by the accompanying gliosis, while in infracted areas, the diffusion trace approaches that of free water and may hence be higher than that in areas of WMC. Furthermore, loss of ordered axonal tracts and the accompanying non-directionally orientated gliosis result in marked loss of FA.

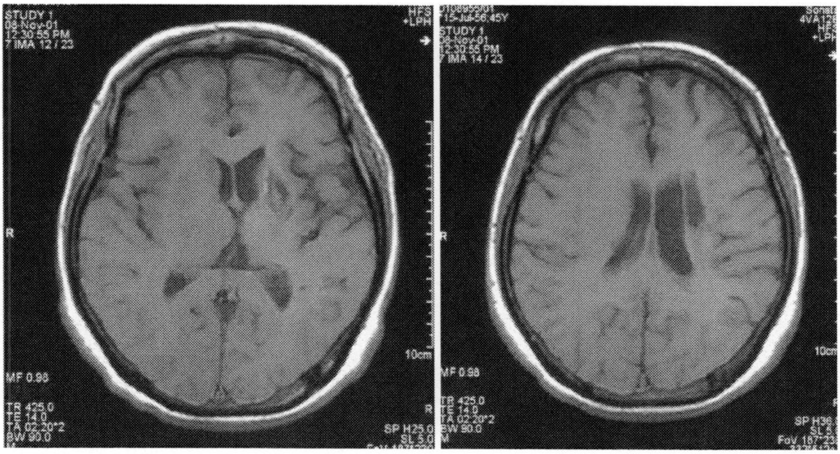

Figure 3. A case of poststroke vascular dementia not fulfilling NINDS-AIREN imaging criteria

The patient is a 45-year-old woman with poststroke dementia. Her dementia developed within 3 months after the stroke episode. At 1 year poststroke, she had residual mild expressive aphasia, poor attention span, anterograde memory loss, emotional lability, and depression. Her MMSE was 19/30. T1-weighted MRI shows left lentiform nucleus infarct (left) extending to the left corona radiata (right) with compensatory dilation of the lateral ventricle. MRA (not shown) showed severe stenosis of the left MCA. Even though the patient clearly had poststroke VaD, she was excluded from a multi-center drug trial, as her imaging features do not fulfill the imaging criteria of NINDS-AIREN.

O'Sullivan demonstrated recently that diffusion tensor measures (mean diffusivity and FA) on normal appearing white matter among patients with lacunar stroke correlated significantly with executive dysfunction, while measures of lesions (WMC and lacunar infarcts) volume on conventional T1-weighted and FLAIR did not correlate with executive dysfunction [156]. These findings probably suggest that DTI measure for white matter structural abnormality is more sensitive and at the same time more specific than conventional MRI. Interestingly, DTI measures in region of WMC as demonstrated by conventional MRI did not correlate with cognitive measures. Similar findings were also noted in patients with CADASIL by the same group of investigators [157]. A recent longitudinal study using DTI techniques (diffusion trace histograms analyses for the whole brain) also demonstrated its usefulness in monitoring progression of tissue damage among CADASIL patients [158]. Further study is needed to evaluate the correlation between cognitive deterioration and changes in DTI measures over time and its role as a surrogate marker in clinical trials [88]. Note that recent advances in DTI techniques have made fiber-tracking possible and 3 dimensional anatomical details of white matter fibers can be reconstructed via appropriate software programs. Yet its role in the evaluation of PSD needs further research.

Magnetization Transfer Imaging

Similar to DTI, MTI technique aims also to measure tissue integrity with greater specificity than conventional MRI. Contrast on MTI is based upon interactions between "free" water protons and protons "bound" to macromolecules, e.g. myelin. By using a special off-resonance pulse, which saturates the magnetization of bound protons, magnetization will also be transferred from the free to the bound protons, thus reducing the magnetic resonance signal. Tissue integrity is related to measure of the bound protons. The magnetization transfer data are commonly quantified as the magnetization transfer ratio (MTR), which is obtained by dividing the signal intensities in the region of interest without a magnetization transfer prepulse by those with such a prepulse and multiply by 100. Tissue damage (e.g. ischemic WMC) is reflected by a low MTR, which implies the incapability of macromolecules to exchange magnetization with free water protons.

Although MTI has been used mainly in the study of WMC associated with multiple sclerosis, it has also been recently applied in those with cerebral SVD and CADASIL.[159, 160] Among patients with SVD and normal subjects, although MTR of total MRI visible WMC and non-periventricular WMC were similar between the two groups, MTR of periventricular WMC were significantly lower in patients than that in controls.[160] This suggested that myelin loss might probably be more severe in periventricular WMC relative to other regions of WMC. In another recent study among CADASIL patients, MTR was not only lower in the MRI visible WMC, but was also lower in the normal appearing white and gray matter. Moreover, MTR from all tissues (apart from normal appearing gray matter) were found to correlate with age, physical disability, and cognitive impairment [159]. Overall, these initial findings suggest that similar to DTI, MTI and MTR may be more specific for pathological white matter damage and more sensitive for detection of early disease changes.

$T2^*$-Weighted GE (Figure 2e)

The superiority of $T2^*$-weighted GE sequence over basic SE sequence in detection of microbleeds has been established. Microbleed is associated with ICH, SVD, stroke patients, hypertensive elderly, CADASIL, or CAA. Microbleed is currently believed to be a manifestation of small arterial damage, in which minimal blood leaks through damaged small artery. Its presence may not only reflect severity of SVD, [161] more importantly, it may predict development of intracerebral bleeding with use of antithrombotic and thrombolytic treatments. Werring et al recently demonstrated that among stroke patients, number and location (basal ganglia and frontal lobes) of microbleeds visible on $T2^*$-weighted GE images correlated significantly with executive dysfunction independent of the extent of WMC.[68] Further study is needed to confirm its relevance to PSD.

Magnetic Resonance Perfusion

In previous section, the role of PET, SPECT, and xenon CT in elucidating the ischemic origin of WMC by demonstrating reduced CBF at regions of subcortical ischemic lesions had been mentioned. However, there are certain limitations with these standard functional imaging modalities. First, such techniques require exposure to radioactive substance. Second, only semi-quantitative measurements can be obtained by SPECT. Third, poor spatial resolution with these modalities and need of co-registration of PET or SPECT images to MRI/CT, hence making delineation between normal appearing white matter and WMC overall difficult. Recent advance in MRI has now made it possible to perform quantification of CBF using exogenous contrast-based perfusion MRI along with high spatial resolution. This technique was recently applied in the evaluation of WMC among patients with lacunar stroke by O'Sullivan et al. [162]. This study demonstrated clearly that not only CBF was reduced in WMC relative to normal appearing white matter, it was also reduced in normal appearing periventricular white matter among stroke patients relative to that in controls. It will be of paramount importance to investigate whether presence of reduced CBF at normal appearing white matter predicts development of actual WMC, and if that occurs, to further explore therapy that can reverse this perfusion deficit and /or development of WMC.

Magnetic Resonance Spectroscopy (Figure 2h)

In vivo MRS measures the regional distribution of important metabolites (e.g. N-acetylaspartate [NAA], myo-inositol, creatine [Cr], choline [Cho]-containing compounds) in the brain. Similar to standard functional studies, it can reveal abnormalities that are not visible on structural imaging, and hence can help to understand the mechanisms of cognitive impairment in stroke or differentiation between dementias. It has been increasingly used particularly in the evaluation of cognitive impairment associated with cerebral SVD in recent years [163, 164]. Using proton (^{1}H) MRS, Capizzano et el demonstrated that patients with dementia and lacunaes had reduced NAA not only in white matter region, but also in gray matter region relative to healthy controls [163]. In another study, Schuff et al also demonstrated that patients with SVD had lower NAA in frontal cortex and left parietal cortex relative to that in AD patients and cortical NAA was noted to decrease with increasing WMC and number of lacunes. In the same study, adding parietal NAA to MRI-derived hippocampal atrophy improved separation between SVD and AD from 79% to 89%. This study with MRS confirms the importance of cortical dysfunction associated with subcortical ischemic lesions and suggests a characteristic pattern of metabolite change that may serve as a basis for improved diagnosis.

L. Take-Home-Messages

Poststroke dementia has been a neglected area although it is common, disabling, and potentially preventable. Different to AD, which is a homogeneous entity, PSD is heterogeneous with complexity far exceeds that of AD or the traditional concept of multi-infarct dementia. Findings from imaging studies have contributed significantly to our present understanding and management of PSD. It is currently believed that PSD may involve complex interactions between vascular etiologies, vascular related brain lesions, brain atrophy, co-existing dementing diseases, host factors, and vascular risk factors. At present, potential treatments depend on its underlying vascular etiology and etiology of dementia; hence, we propose to classify PSD according to these two factors. Basic imaging modalities for the evaluation of PSD are CT and MRI (T1-, T2-, and PD weighted and FLAIR), which can provide relevant imaging variables including vascular related brain lesions (e.g. size, site, laterality, multiplicity, pattern), extent of WMC, and brain atrophy (cortical, subcortical, general, regional). Common imaging variables that predict poststroke VaD include size of left sided anterior corona radiata infarct and extent of WMC. Lesions at other strategic sites (e.g. thalamus, genu of internal capsule, angular gyrus) causing poststroke VaD are generally less common. Although atrophy measures appear to affect cognition more than ischemic measures (WMC and lacunar infarcts) in lacunar stroke, cortical and callosal atrophy correlates with extent of WMC. Findings from xenon CT, PET, and SPECT have also contributed to our understanding of the pathophysiology of WMC and mechanisms of dementia in PSD. Although it is also able to differentiate between different etiologies of dementia, its cost, complexity, and inconvenience have limited its clinical utility. The NINDS-AIREN criteria incorporate the most detailed imaging criteria to aid the diagnosis of VaD, yet modification is needed to improve its sensitivity and inter-rater agreement. Recent applications of more advanced MRI techniques including DWI, DTI, MTI, MR perfusion, and MRS, have enhanced early detection of ischemic brain tissue with increased specificity, better understanding on the pathophysiology of WMC, and/or our ability to differentiate between various etiologies of dementia in PSD. Further study is warranted to evaluate the usefulness of imaging variables (e.g. progression of WMC and cerebral perfusion and metabolism) as surrogate markers in clinical trials.

Appendix

Commonly Used Visual Scales for Rating Severity of WMC

1. Fazekas and Schmidt Scale [109]

White matter hyperintensity (WMH)

(0) Absent
(1) Punctate
(2) Beginning confluent
(3) Confluent or irregular periventricular hyperintensities

2. The Scheltens Scale [111]

Periventricular hyperintensities (PVH 0-6)		
Caps: occipital	0 /1 /2	0 = absent
Frontal	0 /1 /2	1 = ≤ 5mm
Bands: lat. Ventricles	0 /1 /2	2 = > 5mm and < 10 mm
White matter hyperintensities (WMH 0-24)		
Frontal	0 /1 /2 /3 /4 /5 /6	0 = n.a.
Parietal	0 /1 /2 /3 /4 /5 /6	1 = < 3 mm; n ≤ 5
Occipital	0 /1 /2 /3 /4 /5 /6	2 = < 3 mm; n > 6
Temporal	0 /1 /2 /3 /4 /5 /6	3 = 4-10 mm; n ≤ 5
		4 = 4 mm, n > 6
		5 = > 11 mm; n > 1
		6 = confluent

2. The Scheltens Scale [111] (Continued)

Basal ganglia hyperintensities (BG 0-30)	
Caudate Nucleus	0 /1 /2 /3 /4 /5 /6
Putamen	0 /1 /2 /3 /4 /5 /6
Globus Pallidus	0 /1 /2 /3 /4 /5 /6
Thalamus	0 /1 /2 /3 /4 /5 /6
Internal capsule	0 /1 /2 /3 /4 /5 /6
Infra-tentorial foci of hyperintensity (ITF 0-24)	
Cerebellum	0 /1 /2 /3 /4 /5 /6
Mesencephalon	0 /1 /2 /3 /4 /5 /6
Pons	0 /1 /2 /3 /4 /5 /6
Medulla	0 /1 /2 /3 /4 /5 /6

Semiquantative rating of signal hyperintensities in separate regions, with the range of the scale, between brackets. n = number of lesions; n.a. = no abnormalities.

3. The Age Related WMC Rating Scale for MRI or CT [95]

White matter lesions	
0	No lesions (including symmetrical, well-defined caps or bands)
1	Focal lesions
2	Beginning confluence of lesions
3	Without involvement of U fibers
Basal ganglia lesions	
0	No lesions
1	1 focal lesion (≥5mm)
2	>1 focal lesion
3	Confluent lesions

White matter changes on MRI were defined as bright lesions ≥5mm on T2, PD, or FLAIR images. Lesions on CT were defined as hypodense areas of ≥5mm; left and right hemispheres were rated separately. The following brain areas were used for rating: frontal, parieto-occipital, temporal, infratentorial/cerebellum, and basal ganglia (striatum, globus pallidus, thalamus, internal/external capsule, and insula).

References

[1] Ivan CS, Seshadri S, Beiser A, et al. Dementia after stroke: the Framingham Study. *Stroke* 2004; 35:1264-8.

[2] Tatemichi TK, Desmond DW, Mayeux R, et al. Dementia after stroke: baseline frequency, risks, and clinical features in a hospitalized cohort. *Neurology* 1992; 42:1185-93.

[3] Tatemichi TK, Paik M, Bagiella E, et al. Risk of dementia after stroke in a hospitalized cohort: results of a longitudinal study. *Neurology* 1994; 44:1885-91.

[4] Desmond DW, Moroney JT, Sano M, et al. Incidence of dementia after ischemic stroke: results of a longitudinal study. *Stroke* 2002; 33:2254-60.

[5] Zhou DH, Wang JY, Li J, et al. Study on frequency and predictors of dementia after ischemic strokeThe Chongqing Stroke Study. *J. Neurol.* 2004; 251:421-7.

[6] Chiu HF, Lam LC, Chi I, et al. Prevalence of dementia in Chinese elderly in Hong Kong. *Neurology* 1998; 50:1002-9.

[7] Lobo A, Launer LJ, Fratiglioni L, et al. Prevalence of dementia and major subtypes in Europe: A collaborative study of population-based cohorts. Neurologic Diseases in the Elderly Research Group. *Neurology* 2000; 54:S4-9.

[8] Moroney JT, Bagiella E, Tatemichi TK, et al. Dementia after stroke increases the risk of long-term stroke recurrence. *Neurology* 1997; 48:1317-25.

[9] Desmond DW, Moroney JT, Sano M, et al. Mortality in patients with dementia after ischemic stroke. *Neurology* 2002; 59:537-43.

[10] Barba R, Morin MD, Cemillan C, et al. Previous and incident dementia as risk factors for mortality in stroke patients. *Stroke* 2002; 33:1993-8.

[11] Sachdev PS, Brodaty H, Valenzuela MJ, et al. The neuropsychological profile of vascular cognitive impairment in stroke and TIA patients. *Neurology* 2004; 62:912-9.

[12] Pohjasvaara T, Leskela M, Vataja R, et al. Post-stroke depression, executive dysfunction and functional outcome. *Eur. J. Neurol.* 2002; 9:269-75.

[13] Tatemichi TK, Desmond DW, Stern Y, et al. Cognitive impairment after stroke: frequency, patterns, and relationship to functional abilities. *J. Neurol. Neurosurg. Psychiatry* 1994; 57:202-7.

[14] Mok VCT, Wong A, Lam WWM, et al. Cognitive impairment and functional outcome after stroke associated with small vessel disease. *J. Neurol. Neurosurg. Psychiatry* 2004:560-566.

[15] Hachinski VC, Lassen NA, Marshall J. Multi-infarct dementia. A cause of mental deterioration in the elderly. *Lancet* 1974; 2:207-10.

[16] Roman GC, Tatemichi TK, Erkinjuntti T, et al. Vascular dementia: diagnostic criteria for research studies. Report of the NINDS-AIREN International Workshop. *Neurology* 1993; 43:250-60.

[17] Pohjasvaara T, Mantyla R, Salonen O, et al. How complex interactions of ischemic brain infarcts, white matter lesions, and atrophy relate to poststroke dementia. *Arch. Neurol.* 2000; 57:1295-300.

[18] Altieri M, Di Piero V, Pasquini M, et al. Delayed poststroke dementia: a 4-year follow-up study. *Neurology* 2004; 62:2193-7.

[19] Henon H, Durieu I, Guerouaou D, et al. Poststroke dementia: incidence and relationship to prestroke cognitive decline. *Neurology* 2001; 57:1216-22.

[20] Hachinski VC, Iliff LD, Zilhka E, et al. Cerebral blood flow in dementia. *Arch. Neurol.* 1975; 32:632-7.

[21] Association AP. *Diagnostic and statistical manual disorders*: Washington, DC, 1994.

[22] Organization. WH. ICD-10 Classification of Mental and Behavioural Disorders: *Diagnostic Criteria for Research*. Geneva; WHO, 1993.

[23] Chui HC, Victoroff JI, Margolin D, et al. Criteria for the diagnosis of ischemic vascular dementia proposed by the State of California Alzheimer's Disease Diagnostic and Treatment Centers. *Neurology* 1992; 42:473-80.

[24] Pohjasvaara T, Mantyla R, Ylikoski R, et al. Comparison of different clinical criteria (DSM-III, ADDTC, ICD-10, NINDS-AIREN, DSM-IV) for the diagnosis of vascular dementia. National Institute of Neurological Disorders and Stroke-Association Internationale pour la Recherche et l'Enseignement en Neurosciences. *Stroke* 2000; 31:2952-7.

[25] Gold G, Giannakopoulos P, Montes-Paixao Junior C, et al. Sensitivity and specificity of newly proposed clinical criteria for possible vascular dementia. *Neurology* 1997; 49:690-4.

[26] Erkinjuntti T, Inzitari D, Pantoni L, et al. Research criteria for subcortical vascular dementia in clinical trials. *J. Neural. Transm. Suppl.* 2000; 59:23-30.

[27] Meyer JS, Xu G, Thornby J, et al. Is mild cognitive impairment prodromal for vascular dementia like Alzheimer's disease? *Stroke* 2002; 33:1981-5.

[28] Feinberg TE, Rothi LJ, Heilman KM. Multimodal agnosia after unilateral left hemisphere lesion. *Neurology* 1986; 36:864-7.

[29] Kertesz A, Ferro JM, Shewan CM. Apraxia and aphasia: the functional-anatomical basis for their dissociation. *Neurology* 1984; 34:40-7.

[30] Van Zandvoort MJ, Kappelle LJ, Algra A, et al. Decreased capacity for mental effort after single supratentorial lacunar infarct may affect performance in everyday life. *J. Neurol. Neurosurg. Psychiatry* 1998; 65:697-702.

[31] Rockwood K, Wentzel C, Hachinski V, et al. Prevalence and outcomes of vascular cognitive impairment. Vascular Cognitive Impairment Investigators of the Canadian Study of Health and Aging. *Neurology* 2000; 54:447-51.

[32] Mok VC, Fan YH, Lam WW, et al. Small subcortical infarct and intracranial large artery disease in Chinese. *J. Neurol. Sci.* 2003; 216:55-9.

[33] Wong KS, Gao S, Chan YL, et al. Mechanisms of acute cerebral infarctions in patients with middle cerebral artery stenosis: a diffusion-weighted imaging and microemboli monitoring study. *Ann. Neurol.* 2002; 52:74-81.

[34] Mendez MF, Adams NL, Lewandowski KS. Neurobehavioral changes associated with caudate lesions. *Neurology* 1989; 39:349-54.

[35] Auchus AP, Chen CP, Sodagar SN, et al. Single stroke dementia: insights from 12 cases in Singapore. *J. Neurol. Sci.* 2002; 203-204:85-9.

[36] Tatemichi TK, Desmond DW, Prohovnik I, et al. Confusion and memory loss from capsular genu infarction: a thalamocortical disconnection syndrome? *Neurology* 1992; 42:1966-79.

[37] Bhatia KP, Marsden CD. The behavioural and motor consequences of focal lesions of the basal ganglia in man. *Brain* 1994; 117 (Pt 4):859-76.

[38] Babikian V, Ropper AH. Binswanger's disease: a review. *Stroke* 1987; 18:2-12.

[39] Ishii N, Nishihara Y, Imamura T. Why do frontal lobe symptoms predominate in vascular dementia with lacunes? *Neurology* 1986; 36:340-5.

[40] Roman GC, Erkinjuntti T, Wallin A, et al. Subcortical ischaemic vascular dementia. *Lancet Neurol.* 2002; 1:426-36.

[41] Mori S, Sadoshima S, Ibayashi S, et al. Impact of thalamic hematoma on six-month mortality and motor and cognitive functional outcome. *Stroke* 1995; 26:620-6.

[42] Szirmai I, Vastagh I, Szombathelyi E, et al. Strategic infarcts of the thalamus in vascular dementia. *J. Neurol. Sci.* 2002; 203-204:91-7.

[43] Bugiani O. A beta-related cerebral amyloid angiopathy. *Neurol. Sci.* 2004; 25 Suppl 1:S1-2.

[44] Gray F, Dubas F, Roullet E, Escourolle R. Leukoencephalopathy in diffuse hemorrhagic cerebral amyloid angiopathy. *Ann. Neurol.* 1985; 18:54-9.

[45] Olichney JM, Hansen LA, Hofstetter CR, et al. Association between severe cerebral amyloid angiopathy and cerebrovascular lesions in Alzheimer disease is not a spurious one attributable to apolipoprotein E4. *Arch. Neurol.* 2000; 57:869-74.

[46] Dichgans M. Cerebral autosomal dominant arteriopathy with subcortical infarcts and leukoencephalopathy: phenotypic and mutational spectrum. *J. Neurol. Sci*. 2002; 203-204:77-80.

[47] Tatemichi TK, Foulkes MA, Mohr JP, et al. Dementia in stroke survivors in the Stroke Data Bank cohort. Prevalence, incidence, risk factors, and computed tomographic findings. *Stroke* 1990; 21:858-66.

[48] Desmond DW, Moroney JT, Paik MC, et al. Frequency and clinical determinants of dementia after ischemic stroke. *Neurology* 2000; 54:1124-31.

[49] Pohjasvaara T, Erkinjuntti T, Ylikoski R, et al. Clinical determinants of poststroke dementia. *Stroke* 1998; 29:75-81.

[50] Tang WK, Chan SS, Chiu HF, et al. Frequency and determinants of poststroke dementia in Chinese. *Stroke* 2004; 35:930-5.

[51] Henon H, Pasquier F, Durieu I, et al. Preexisting dementia in stroke patients. Baseline frequency, associated factors, and outcome. *Stroke* 1997; 28:2429-36.

[52] Barba R, Castro MD, del Mar Morin M, et al. Prestroke dementia. *Cerebrovasc. Dis*. 2001; 11:216-24.

[53] Snowdon DA, Greiner LH, Mortimer JA, et al. Brain infarction and the clinical expression of Alzheimer disease. The Nun Study. *Jama* 1997; 277:813-7.

[54] Esiri MM, Nagy Z, Smith MZ, et al. Cerebrovascular disease and threshold for dementia in the early stages of Alzheimer's disease. *Lancet* 1999; 354:919-20.

[55] Mobius HJ, Stoffler A. New approaches to clinical trials in vascular dementia: memantine in small vessel disease. *Cerebrovasc. Dis*. 2002; 13 Suppl 2:61-6.

[56] Pantoni L, Rossi R, Inzitari D, et al. Efficacy and safety of nimodipine in subcortical vascular dementia: a subgroup analysis of the Scandinavian Multi-Infarct Dementia Trial. *J. Neurol. Sci.* 2000; 175:124-34.

[57] Erkinjuntti T, Kurz A, Gauthier S, et al. Efficacy of galantamine in probable vascular dementia and Alzheimer's disease combined with cerebrovascular disease: a randomised trial. *Lancet* 2002; 359:1283-90.

[58] Mirra SS, Heyman A, McKeel D, et al. The Consortium to Establish a Registry for Alzheimer's Disease (CERAD). Part II. Standardization of the neuropathologic assessment of Alzheimer's disease. *Neurology* 1991; 41:479-86.

[59] Jellinger KA. The pathology of ischemic-vascular dementia: an update. *J. Neurol. Sci.* 2002; 203-204:153-7.

[60] Erkinjuntti T, Haltia M, Palo J, et al. Accuracy of the clinical diagnosis of vascular dementia: a prospective clinical and post-mortem neuropathological study. *J. Neurol. Neurosurg. Psychiatry* 1988; 51:1037-44.

[61] White L, Petrovitch H, Hardman J, et al. Cerebrovascular pathology and dementia in autopsied Honolulu-Asia Aging Study participants. *Ann. NY Acad. Sci.* 2002; 977:9-23.

[62] Fazekas F, Kleinert R, Roob G, et al. Histopathologic analysis of foci of signal loss on gradient-echo T2*-weighted MR images in patients with spontaneous intracerebral hemorrhage: evidence of microangiopathy-related microbleeds. *AJNR Am. J. Neuroradiol.* 1999; 20:637-42.

[63] Kalaria RN, Kenny RA, Ballard CG, et al. Towards defining the neuropathological substrates of vascular dementia. *J. Neurol. Sci.* 2004; 226:75-80.

[64] Lammie GA. Pathology of lacunar infarction. In: Donnan GA, Norrving, B., Bamford, J.M., Bogousslavsky, J., ed. *Subcortical stroke*. Oxford: Oxford University Press, 2002:37-46.

[65] Wardlaw JM, Sandercock PA, Dennis MS, et al. Is breakdown of the blood-brain barrier responsible for lacunar stroke, leukoaraiosis, and dementia? *Stroke* 2003; 34:806-12.

[66] Moody DM, Brown WR, Challa VR, et al. Periventricular venous collagenosis: association with leukoaraiosis. *Radiology* 1995; 194:469-76.

[67] Fazekas F, Kleinert R, Offenbacher H, et al. Pathologic correlates of incidental MRI white matter signal hyperintensities. *Neurology* 1993; 43:1683-9.

[68] Werring DJ, Frazer DW, Coward LJ, et al. Cognitive dysfunction in patients with cerebral microbleeds on T2*-weighted gradient-echo MRI. *Brain* 2004; 127:2265-75.

[69] Barba R, Martinez-Espinosa S, Rodriguez-Garcia E, et al. Poststroke dementia : clinical features and risk factors. *Stroke* 2000; 31:1494-501.

[70] Tatemichi TK, Desmond DW, Paik M, et al. Clinical determinants of dementia related to stroke. *Ann. Neurol.* 1993; 33:568-75.

[71] Klimkowicz A, Dziedzic T, Slowik A, et al. Incidence of pre- and poststroke dementia: cracow stroke registry. *Dement. Geriatr. Cogn. Disord.* 2002; 14:137-40.

[72] Lin JH, Lin RT, Tai CT, et al. Prediction of poststroke dementia. *Neurology* 2003; 61:343-8.

[73] Censori B, Manara O, Agostinis C, et al. Dementia after first stroke. *Stroke* 1996; 27:1205-10.

[74] Pohjasvaara T, Erkinjuntti T, Vataja R, et al. Dementia three months after stroke. Baseline frequency and effect of different definitions of dementia in the Helsinki Stroke Aging Memory Study (SAM) cohort. *Stroke* 1997; 28:785-92.

[75] Inzitari D, Di Carlo A, Pracucci G, et al. Incidence and determinants of poststroke dementia as defined by an informant interview method in a hospital-based stroke registry. *Stroke* 1998; 29:2087-93.

[76] Kokmen E, Whisnant JP, O'Fallon WM, et al. Dementia after ischemic stroke: a population-based study in Rochester, Minnesota (1960-1984). Neurology 1996; 46:154-9.

[77] Moroney JT, Tang MX, Berglund L, et al. Low-density lipoprotein cholesterol and the risk of dementia with stroke. *Jama* 1999; 282:254-60.

[78] Cummings JL. Frontal-subcortical circuits and human behavior. *Arch. Neurol.* 1993; 50:873-80.

[79] Royall DR, Lauterbach EC, Cummings JL, et al. Executive control function: a review of its promise and challenges for clinical research. A report from the Committee on Research of the American Neuropsychiatric Association. *J. Neuropsychiatry. Clin. Neurosci.* 2002; 14:377-405.

[80] Tierney MC, Black SE, Szalai JP, et al. Recognition memory and verbal fluency differentiate probable Alzheimer disease from subcortical ischemic vascular dementia. *Arch. Neurol.* 2001; 58:1654-9.

[81] Ballard C, Rowan E, Stephens S, et al. Prospective follow-up study between 3 and 15 months after stroke: improvements and decline in cognitive function among dementia-free stroke survivors >75 years of age. *Stroke* 2003; 34:2440-4.

[82] Sachdev PS, Brodaty H, Valenzuela MJ, et al. Progression of cognitive impairment in stroke patients. *Neurology* 2004; 63:1618-23.

[83] Nyenhuis DL, Gorelick PB, Freels S, et al. Cognitive and functional decline in African Americans with VaD, AD, and stroke without dementia. *Neurology* 2002; 58:56-61.

[84] Pullicino P, Benedict RH, Capruso DX, et al. Neuroimaging criteria for vascular dementia. *Arch. Neurol.* 1996; 53:723-8.

[85] Auchus AP, Brashear HR, Titusville NJ, et al. Results of a trial of galantamine in subjects with vascular dementia confirmed by central MRI reading. *56th Annual Meeting of the American Academy of Neurology* (abstract) 2004.

[86] Mungas D, Reed BR, Jagust WJ, et al. Volumetric MRI predicts rate of cognitive decline related to AD and cerebrovascular disease. *Neurology* 2002; 59:867-73.

[87] De Reuck J, Decoo D, Marchau M, et al. Positron emission tomography in vascular dementia. *J. Neurol. Sci.* 1998; 154:55-61.

[88] Schmidt R, Scheltens P, Erkinjuntti T, et al. White matter lesion progression: a surrogate endpoint for trials in cerebral small-vessel disease. *Neurology* 2004; 63:139-44.

[89] Jobst KA, Smith AD, Szatmari M, et al. Detection in life of confirmed Alzheimer's disease using a simple measurement of medial temporal lobe atrophy by computed tomography. *Lancet* 1992; 340:1179-83.

[90] DeCarli C, Kaye JA, Horwitz B, et al. Critical analysis of the use of computer-assisted transverse axial tomography to study human brain in aging and dementia of the Alzheimer type. *Neurology* 1990; 40:872-83.

[91] Broderick JP, Brott TG, Grotta JC. Intracerebral hemorrhage volume measurement. *Stroke* 1994; 25:1081.

[92] Kawamura J, Meyer JS, Terayama Y, et al. Cerebral hypoperfusion correlates with mild and parenchymal loss with severe multi-infarct dementia. J Neurol Sci 1991; 102:32-8.

[93] Gorelick PB, Chatterjee A, Patel D, et al. Cranial computed tomographic observations in multi-infarct dementia. A controlled study. *Stroke* 1992; 23:804-11.

[94] Wahlund LO, Barkhof F, Fazekas F, et al. A new rating scale for age-related white matter changes applicable to MRI and CT. Stroke 2001; 32:1318-22.

[95] Loeb C, Gandolfo C, Croce R, et al. Dementia associated with lacunar infarction. *Stroke* 1992; 23:1225-9.

[96] van Swieten JC, Hijdra A, Koudstaal PJ, et al. Grading white matter lesions on CT and MRI: a simple scale. *J. Neurol. Neurosurg. Psychiatry* 1990; 53:1080-3.

[97] Pantoni L, Garcia JH. The significance of cerebral white matter abnormalities 100 years after Binswanger's report. A review. *Stroke* 1995; 26:1293-301.

[98] Geroldi C, Galluzzi S, Testa C, et al. Validation study of a CT-based weighted rating scale for subcortical ischemic vascular disease in patients with mild cognitive deterioration. *Eur. Neurol.* 2003; 49:193-209.

[99] Albert M, Naeser MA, Levine HL, et al. Ventricular size in patients with presenile dementia of the Alzheimer's type. *Arch. Neurol.* 1984; 41:1258-63.

[100] Victoroff J, Mack WJ, Grafton ST, et al. A method to improve interrater reliability of visual inspection of brain MRI scans in dementia. *Neurology* 1994; 44:2267-76.

[101] Hughes CP, Gado M. Computed tomography and aging of the brain. *Radiology* 1981; 139:391-6.

[102] Damasio H, Eslinger P, Damasio AR, et al. Quantitative computed tomographic analysis in the diagnosis of dementia. *Arch. Neurol.* 1983; 40:715-9.

[103] Turkheimer E, Cullum CM, Hubler DW, et al. Quantifying cortical atrophy. *J. Neurol. Neurosurg. Psychiatry* 1984; 47:1314-8.

[104] Bokura H, Kobayashi S, Yamaguchi S. Distinguishing silent lacunar infarction from enlarged Virchow-Robin spaces: a magnetic resonance imaging and pathological study. *J. Neurol.* 1998; 245:116-22.

[105] Mantyla R, Aronen HJ, Salonen O, et al. The prevalence and distribution of white-matter changes on different MRI pulse sequences in a post-stroke cohort. *Neuroradiology* 1999; 41:657-65.

[106] Herskovits EH, Itoh R, Melhem ER. Accuracy for detection of simulated lesions: comparison of fluid-attenuated inversion-recovery, proton density--weighted, and T2-weighted synthetic brain MR imaging. *AJR Am. J. Roentgenol.* 2001; 176:1313-8.

[107] Manolio TA, Kronmal RA, Burke GL, et al. Magnetic resonance abnormalities and cardiovascular disease in older adults. The Cardiovascular Health Study. *Stroke* 1994; 25:318-27.

[108] Schmidt R, Fazekas F, Kleinert G, et al. Magnetic resonance imaging signal hyperintensities in the deep and subcortical white matter. A comparative

study between stroke patients and normal volunteers. *Arch. Neurol.* 1992; 49:825-7.

[109] de Groot JC, de Leeuw FE, Oudkerk M, et al. Cerebral white matter lesions and cognitive function: the Rotterdam Scan Study. *Ann. Neurol.* 2000; 47:145-51.

[110] Scheltens P, Barkhof F, Leys D, et al. A semiquantative rating scale for the assessment of signal hyperintensities on magnetic resonance imaging. *J. Neurol. Sci.* 1993; 114:7-12.

[111] Mantyla R, Erkinjuntti T, Salonen O, et al. Variable agreement between visual rating scales for white matter hyperintensities on MRI. Comparison of 13 rating scales in a poststroke cohort. *Stroke* 1997; 28:1614-23.

[112] Prins ND, van Straaten EC, van Dijk EJ, et al. Measuring progression of cerebral white matter lesions on MRI: visual rating and volumetrics. *Neurology* 2004; 62:1533-9.

[113] Fan YH, Lam WW, Mok VC, et al. Variability and validity of a simple visual rating scale in grading white matter changes on magnetic resonance imaging. *J. Neuroimaging.* 2003; 13:255-8.

[114] Kapeller P, Barber R, Vermeulen RJ, et al. Visual rating of age-related white matter changes on magnetic resonance imaging: scale comparison, interrater agreement, and correlations with quantitative measurements. *Stroke* 2003; 34:441-5.

[115] Fein G, Di Sclafani V, Tanabe J, et al. Hippocampal and cortical atrophy predict dementia in subcortical ischemic vascular disease. *Neurology* 2000; 55:1626-35.

[116] Scheltens P, Leys D, Barkhof F, et al. Atrophy of medial temporal lobes on MRI in "probable" Alzheimer's disease and normal ageing: diagnostic value and neuropsychological correlates. *J. Neurol. Neurosurg. Psychiatry* 1992; 55:967-72.

[117] Yamauchi H, Fukuyama H, Shio H. Corpus callosum atrophy in patients with leukoaraiosis may indicate global cognitive impairment. *Stroke* 2000; 31:1515-20.

[118] Bigler ED, Neeley ES, Miller MJ, et al. Cerebral volume loss, cognitive deficit and neuropsychological performance: comparative measures of brain atrophy: I. Dementia. *J. Int. Neuropsychol. Soc.* 2004; 10:442-52.

[119] Coffey CE, Wilkinson WE, Parashos IA, et al. Quantitative cerebral anatomy of the aging human brain: a cross-sectional study using magnetic resonance imaging. *Neurology* 1992; 42:527-36.

[120] O'Brien JT, Paling S, Barber R, et al. Progressive brain atrophy on serial MRI in dementia with Lewy bodies, AD, and vascular dementia. *Neurology* 2001; 56:1386-8.

[121] Liu CK, Miller BL, Cummings JL, et al. A quantitative MRI study of vascular dementia. *Neurology* 1992; 42:138-43.

[122] Starkstein SE, Sabe L, Vazquez S, et al. Neuropsychological, psychiatric, and cerebral blood flow findings in vascular dementia and Alzheimer's disease. *Stroke* 1996; 27:408-14.

[123] Kwan LT, Reed BR, Eberling JL, et al. Effects of subcortical cerebral infarction on cortical glucose metabolism and cognitive function. *Arch. Neurol.* 1999; 56:809-14.

[124] Pappata S, Mazoyer B, Tran Dinh S, et al. Effects of capsular or thalamic stroke on metabolism in the cortex and cerebellum: a positron tomography study. *Stroke* 1990; 21:519-24.

[125] Reed BR, Eberling JL, Mungas D, et al. Frontal lobe hypometabolism predicts cognitive decline in patients with lacunar infarcts. *Arch. Neurol.* 2001; 58:493-7.

[126] Sabri O RE, Hellwig D, Schneider R, et al. Neuropsychological impairment correlates with hypoperfusion and hypometabolism but not with severity of white matter lesions on MRI in patients with cerebral microangiopathy. *Stroke* 1999; 30:556-66.

[127] Yao H, Sadoshima S, Kuwabara Y, et al. Cerebral blood flow and oxygen metabolism in patients with vascular dementia of the Binswanger type. *Stroke* 1990; 21:1694-9.

[128] Rogers RL, Meyer JS, Mortel KF, et al. Decreased cerebral blood flow precedes multi-infarct dementia, but follows senile dementia of Alzheimer type. *Neurology* 1986; 36:1-6.

[129] Reed BR, Eberling JL, Mungas D, et al. Memory failure has different mechanisms in subcortical stroke and Alzheimer's disease. *Ann. Neurol.* 2000; 48:275-84.

[130] Loizou LA, Kendall BE, Marshall J. Subcortical arteriosclerotic encephalopathy: a clinical and radiological investigation. *J. Neurol. Neurosurg. Psychiatry* 1981; 44:294-304.

[131] Pantoni L, Garcia JH. Pathogenesis of leukoaraiosis: a review. *Stroke* 1997; 28:652-9.

[132] De Reuck J, Decoo D, Hasenbroekx MC, et al. Acetazolamide vasoreactivity in vascular dementia: a positron emission tomographic study. *Eur. Neurol.* 1999; 41:31-6.

[133] Mielke R, Kessler J, Szelies B, et al. Vascular dementia: perfusional and metabolic disturbances and effects of therapy. *J. Neural. Transm. Suppl.* 1996; 47:183-91.

[134] Lojkowska W, Ryglewicz D, Jedrzejczak T, et al. The effect of cholinesterase inhibitors on the regional blood flow in patients with Alzheimer's disease and vascular dementia. *J. Neurol. Sci.* 2003; 216:119-26.

[135] Pohjasvaara T, Mantyla R, Salonen O, et al. MRI correlates of dementia after first clinical ischemic stroke. *J. Neurol. Sci.* 2000; 181:111-7.

[136] Cordoliani-Mackowiak MA, Henon H, Pruvo JP, et al. Poststroke dementia: influence of hippocampal atrophy. *Arch. Neurol.* 2003; 60:585-90.

[137] Mungas D, Jagust WJ, Reed BR, et al. MRI predictors of cognition in subcortical ischemic vascular disease and Alzheimer's disease. *Neurology* 2001; 57:2229-35.

[138] Wen HM, Mok VC, Fan YH, et al. Effect of white matter changes on cognitive impairment in patients with lacunar infarcts. *Stroke* 2004; 35:1826-30.

[139] Miyao S, Takano A, Teramoto J, et al. Leukoaraiosis in relation to prognosis for patients with lacunar infarction. *Stroke* 1992; 23:1434-8.

[140] Yamauchi H, Fukuyama H, Ogawa M, et al. Callosal atrophy in patients with lacunar infarction and extensive leukoaraiosis. An indicator of cognitive impairment. *Stroke* 1994; 25:1788-93.

[141] Corbett A, Bennett H, Kos S. Cognitive dysfunction following subcortical infarction. *Arch. Neurol.* 1994; 51:999-1007.

[142] Mok V, Chang C, Wong A, et al. Neuroimaging determinants of cognitive performances in stroke associated with small vessel disease. *Journal of Neuroimaging* 2005; In press.

[143] Dufouil C, Alperovitch A, Tzourio C. Influence of education on the relationship between white matter lesions and cognition. *Neurology* 2003; 60:831-6.

[144] Malm J, Kristensen B, Karlsson T, et al. Cognitive impairment in young adults with infratentorial infarcts. *Neurology* 1998; 51:433-40.

[145] Auer DP, Putz B, Gossl C, et al. Differential lesion patterns in CADASIL and sporadic subcortical arteriosclerotic encephalopathy: MR imaging study with statistical parametric group comparison. *Radiology* 2001; 218:443-51.

[146] Dichgans M, Filippi M, Bruning R, et al. Quantitative MRI in CADASIL: correlation with disability and cognitive performance. *Neurology* 1999; 52:1361-7.

[147] Tatsch K, Koch W, Linke R, et al. Cortical hypometabolism and crossed cerebellar diaschisis suggest subcortically induced disconnection in CADASIL: an 18F-FDG PET study. *J. Nucl. Med.* 2003; 44:862-9.

[148] Vital C, Julien J. Widespread dilatation of perivascular spaces: a leukoencephalopathy causing dementia. *Neurology* 1997; 48:1310-3.

[149] Wetterling T, Kanitz RD, Borgis KJ. Comparison of different diagnostic criteria for vascular dementia (ADDTC, DSM-IV, ICD-10, NINDS-AIREN). *Stroke* 1996; 27:30-6.

[150] van Straaten EC, Scheltens P, Knol DL, et al. Operational definitions for the NINDS-AIREN criteria for vascular dementia: an interobserver study. *Stroke* 2003; 34:1907-12.

[151] Ballard CG, Burton EJ, Barber R, et al. NINDS AIREN neuroimaging criteria do not distinguish stroke patients with and without dementia. *Neurology* 2004; 63:983-8.

[152] Loeb C, Gandolfo C. Diagnostic evaluation of degenerative and vascular dementia. *Stroke* 1983; 14:399-401.

[153] Choi SH, Na DL, Chung CS, et al. Diffusion-weighted MRI in vascular dementia. *Neurology* 2000; 54:83-9.

[154] O'Sullivan M, Rich PM, Barrick TR, et al. Frequency of subclinical lacunar infarcts in ischemic leukoaraiosis and cerebral autosomal dominant arteriopathy with subcortical infarcts and leukoencephalopathy. *AJNR Am. J. Neuroradiol.* 2003; 24:1348-54.

[155] Jones DK, Lythgoe D, Horsfield MA, et al. Characterization of white matter damage in ischemic leukoaraiosis with diffusion tensor MRI. *Stroke* 1999; 30:393-7.

[156] O'Sullivan M, Morris RG, Huckstep B, et al. Diffusion tensor MRI correlates with executive dysfunction in patients with ischaemic leukoaraiosis. *J. Neurol. Neurosurg. Psychiatry* 2004; 75:441-7.

[157] O'Sullivan M, Singhal S, Charlton R, et al. Diffusion tensor imaging of thalamus correlates with cognition in CADASIL without dementia. *Neurology* 2004; 62:702-7.

[158] Molko N, Pappata S, Mangin JF, et al. Monitoring disease progression in CADASIL with diffusion magnetic resonance imaging: a study with whole brain histogram analysis. *Stroke* 2002; 33:2902-8.

[159] Iannucci G, Dichgans M, Rovaris M, et al. Correlations between clinical findings and magnetization transfer imaging metrics of tissue damage in individuals with cerebral autosomal dominant arteriopathy with subcortical infarcts and leukoencephalopathy. *Stroke* 2001; 32:643-8.

[160] Tanabe JL, Ezekiel F, Jagust WJ, et al. Magnetization transfer ratio of white matter hyperintensities in subcortical ischemic vascular dementia. *AJNR Am. J. Neuroradiol.* 1999; 20:839-44.

[161] Fan YH, Mok VC, Lam WW, et al. Cerebral microbleeds and white matter changes in patients hospitalized with lacunar infarcts. *J. Neurol.* 2004; 251:537-41.

[162] O'Sullivan M, Lythgoe DJ, Pereira AC, et al. Patterns of cerebral blood flow reduction in patients with ischemic leukoaraiosis. *Neurology* 2002; 59:321-6.

[163] Capizzano AA, Schuff N, Amend DL, et al. Subcortical ischemic vascular dementia: assessment with quantitative MR imaging and 1H MR spectroscopy. *AJNR Am. J. Neuroradiol.* 2000; 21:621-30.

[164] Schuff N, Capizzano AA, Du AT, et al. Different patterns of N-acetylaspartate loss in subcortical ischemic vascular dementia and AD. *Neurology* 2003; 61:358-64.

Index

A

D

G

H

I

J

L

M

N

O

P

R

S

W

X

Y